FASCIA TRAINING

i

FASCIA TRAINING A WHOLE SYSTEM APPROACH

The New Evidence-Based Science of
Speed, Power, and Injury Resilience

Bill Parisi / Johnathon Allen

Published by Parisi Media Productions

Copyright © 2019

ISBN: 9781797818863

DEDICATED TO my sons, Will and Dan, for being my training subjects and Parisi Speed School models for their entire lives. And my wife, Jennifer, for being my rock and supporting me with all my endeavors. Also, to all of the athletes and coaches around the world who have trained with the Parisi Speed School. Your results and experiences have helped me to continue growing and evolving my own approach to training.

Contents

Forward: A Great Story

WHAT MAKES A GREAT BOOK? There must be an engaging story. It has to be well written and captivating. It must educate and create a platform for application. Fascia Training by Bill Parisi and Johnathon Allen checks all the boxes. The approach they took to gather material for this book was typical of Bill's style. They traveled the country conducting interviews and spending casual time with people who had spent years probing the fascial system and listened to their stories. Along the way, they captured so many seemingly casual comments that added new insight and fostered thought. The magic of a great story occurs when it gives you that *aha!* moment. There are many *aha* moments in the combined synergies of stories pulled out of the different experts interviewed in this book.

Even though I have spoken with Thomas Myers and listened to his lectures, I learned much more from what Bill obtained in the time he spent with Tom. His interviews with legendary Dan Pfaff produced similar gold. I have consulted for Olympic programs internationally, and it is uncanny how many of them mentioned that they had also brought in Dan Pfaff, and that we both had similar foundational thoughts on tuning the body for speed. Ignore the role of fascia at your peril.

In the pursuit of demystifying fascia and its importance for human performance, this book captures the compelling stories and personalities of each expert and their individual journey towards mastery. As one of the people interviewed, I can declare that Bill pulled stories out of me that I had either forgotten or would never think to tell. That is the magic of Parisi and his disarming style. A warm personality who is very likable and engaging, he simply massages the stories out of you, then shares his own insights along the way in a charming *"New Joisy"* style.

I love this book.

– Stu McGill

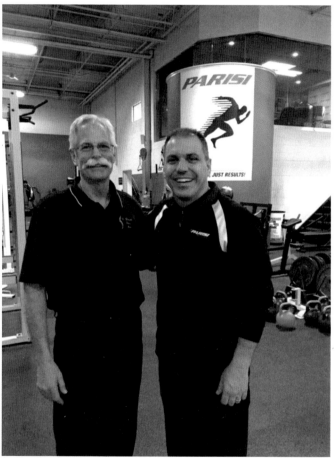

Stu McGill and Bill Parisi at the Parisi Speed School in Fair Lawn, New Jersey.

Bill Parisi / Johnathon Allen

The Quest: An Introduction

TWO INCHES. That was the distance between victory and defeat, between joining the U.S. Junior Track and Field Team in Japan or going home to do whatever it is you do after your dreams of glory and years of training have been crushed in a single decisive moment on the field of competition. This particular moment happened in Chicago the summer after my senior year in high school, where I was competing at the Keebler Junior Invitational Meet for one of two spots as a javelin thrower on the U.S. International Track Team. And lost to a kid who beat me on the last throw of the competition by the length of a golf tee.

After spending the last year of my high school life forgoing the usual senior rites of passage and fun so I could focus entirely on being invited to, and *winning*, that event—becoming New Jersey's top-ranked javelin thrower and one of the top 10 in the country—that aluminum spear felt like it landed squarely in the center of my heart, incinerating it with the heat of a thousand suns. It was the kind of traumatic loss that could have obliterated the competitive spirit of your average teenager. But I was not your average teenager. As I mentally recovered from that most formative of defeats, I used the heat from the atomic blast of those two heart-breaking inches to fuel a new obsession: to seek out the best coaches and training techniques in the world; to unlock the secrets for maximizing power, speed, and athletic performance; and to never experience that feeling again. It was the beginning of a lifelong quest for knowledge that continues to this day.

This quest led me on a search for the top professional coaches of all types, in all areas, starting with acclaimed sports psychologist Dr. Rob Gilbert. "Uncle Rob" helped me focus the searing energy from that loss into a tangible goal that motivated me to attend Iona College, so I could train with Tony Naclerio, the nation's top Olympic javelin coach. While attending Iona, I became a two-time Division 1 All American, qualified for the 1988 Olympic Trials, and set the all-time school record (236',10"). The following year, the quest took me to Finland, where I learned training techniques from the best javelin throwers in the world. At the time, the typical American gym was a sea of selectorized Nautilus weightlifting and cardio equipment, not much different from today's Planet Fitness. I was surprised to find that the Finnish throwers were using very different functional training modalities than I had seen in the States, including dynamic medicine ball drills. I was amazed by how powerful and effective these natural training methods were. It was a mind-blowing paradigm shift in my early athletic education.

After I returned from Finland, I became a graduate assistant in strength and conditioning for the University of Florida Gators Track and Field team, where I continued to study the science of speed and power from the best in the field. I traveled cross country at every opportunity to attend seminars, study with thought leaders, and acquire new knowledge from speed innovators, including Loren Seagrave, Vern Gambetta, Charlie Frances, and Randy Smythe. This quest eventually led me to a presentation by Bulgarian strength coach, Angel Spassov, hosted by NY Giants strength coach, Johnny Parker.

After I impressed Johnny at the event by explaining the functional training and medicine ball techniques I learned in Finland, he offered me a job as an assistant strength and conditioning coach for the New York Giants. It was the opportunity of a lifetime. I began training Super Bowl MVP quarterback Phil Simms on my first day, and we formed an immediate bond. Soon, the skills and training I brought to the program paid off, helping Phil achieve a string of franchise records right up to his final year in the league when he became one of the few quarterbacks in NFL history to start all 16 games of the regular season (winning 11 of them) and was selected to play in the Pro Bowl.

Identifying an emerging opportunity in the marketplace, I opened my first fitness studio in Wyckoff, New Jersey, in 1993—a 3,000-sf space focused exclusively on youth sports performance and speed training. It was the beginning of what would become the Parisi Speed School franchise, which has since grown to include more than 100 locations worldwide—including in China and Saudi Arabia— and trained more than 650,000 athletes between the ages of 7 and 18. Now based at our state-of-the-art flagship facility in Fair Lawn, New Jersey, the Parisi Training System has produced first-round draft picks in every major professional sport—including more than 145 NFL draft picks—and a host of Olympic medalists and champion UFC fighters. In the hands of other like-minded professionals, including renowned martial arts trainer, Martin Rooney, Parisi Training techniques have also served as the foundation for other science-based approaches to optimizing speed, power, and fitness for fighters in the highly successful Training for Warriors program.

Despite all of these achievements, the quest continues. Because, if I've learned anything in the past 25-plus years, it's that if you want better results, you have to be open to new ideas and smarter approaches. You have to be constantly hungry for knowledge. You have to accept that what we don't know about athletic performance and the human body far exceeds what we do know. And that there will always be better, smarter, more efficient ways of training. That's why new world records will always be set. New champions will always emerge. And new techniques and tools will always disrupt the status quo. But to get to that next level, you have to be humble enough to put your existing assumptions aside. And then you need to look at the data, study the science, and interrogate the experts. If all else fails, you have to come up with your own hypothesis and do the research yourself. You have to be that guy (or gal) who discovers the next level. It's part of the beautiful mystery of being human. Every moment is new territory: a fresh opportunity to do things better, faster, smarter.

All it takes is a paradigm shift and an open mind.

What has changed about my quest over the past 25-plus years is that now I'm Bill Parisi. The Brand. The franchise owner. The guy who developed a successful team of coaches and trainers who contribute to a growing list of professional wins and major league championships. And that gives me the opportunity to continue my quest at the highest possible level. Now I get invited to speak at conferences and events around the world alongside many of today's leading experts in sports training and performance, exchanging new knowledge and insights with them along the way.

As a franchise owner, I am constantly being pitched the latest exercise equipment, newfangled gadgets, and training techniques being promoted across the market. And as the leader of a team of coaches, it's incumbent upon me to sort through all of this information to determine what is genuinely new and valid and game-changing and what is—pardon my Jersey French—just marketing bullshit, misconception, and hype.

That puts me in the fortunate position of being able to view a tremendous number of different perspectives from a wide variety of backgrounds that all connect to our ability to improve athletic power, speed, and resilience. What I offer you in this book is an emerging vision for how they all fit together to create a powerful new science-based understanding for unlocking the next evolution in human performance. To be clear, I'm not claiming to be the expert with all the answers. In fact, there's a lot of research and discovery that still needs to be done. And there are a lot of people who know far more than I do about these topics. What I'm saying is that—as I talk to a wide range of professionals from different fields, see the latest technologies, and learn about different techniques from around the globe—I'm beginning to see a new picture emerging for how to improve athletic performance. A true paradigm shift in understanding how the body works. What I'm setting out to do with this book is connect those dots in a way that changes how we think about human power production and athletic potential.

I'm inviting you to join me as we track down and interview thought leaders, including world-renowned anatomy expert and developer of "Anatomy Trains," Thomas Myers; author of multiple books and more than 250 research papers on spinal biomechanics, Stu McGill; and celebrated trainer of national champions and Olympic athletes, Dan Pfaff, and others. We'll look at how new screening tools, like the Sparta Platform™, can deliver deep data that changes our understanding of performance measurement, diagnostics, and injury reduction. And we'll discover how new isokinetic modalities—such as the Delta-Kinetic™ platform developed by OHM Dynamics—are enabling a more integrated, whole-system approach to three-dimensional training that delivers superior results in less time with better injury resilience and faster recovery than the approaches that have gotten us where we are today. No disrespect to the tried and true.

If you don't have the patience for books, I get it. Modern life moves fast. So, here's the 60-second download: Recent studies are showing that our connective tissue network—or "fascia system"—is far more responsible for storing, releasing, and transferring elastic energy through the body than was previously understood, and that three-dimensional, whole-system training of these connective tissues using dynamic natural movements can help athletes achieve better performance while greatly reducing their injury risk.

Data is also showing that the traditional industry focus on training for speed via more strength is often slowing athletes down, and that training the musculoskeletal and cardiovascular systems, without recognizing the significant role the fascia system plays in human movement, increases the risk for injury, especially overuse and connective tissue injuries often seen in basketball, baseball, and running. The best results are achieved using balanced, natural movements with multiple variations in angle, tempo, and load, combined with new diagnostic screening tools that allow trainers to identify where individual deficiencies are, so training can be adjusted accordingly.

But if you have the same hunger for performance; if you want to hear for yourself what the experts have to say, what the data reveals, and what the specific training techniques and modalities are that you can apply to radically improve athletic performance regardless of age, skill level, body type, or sport …. then read on!

The quest continues ….

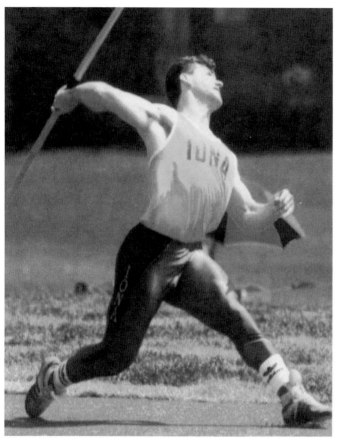

Bill Parisi competing for Iona College circa 1988.

Bill Parisi / Johnathon Allen

Tensegrity: A Balanced Symphony of Systems

CONSIDER FOR A MOMENT that as you sit here reading this book, everything about you is in constant motion. Hold your breath. Sit perfectly still. Pretend to be the statue guy street performer in Times Square, if you want. Your heart is still pumping plasma through your body at an approximate speed of 0.3 meters per second. Electrical impulses fire across your nervous system millions of times per second. Anything you ate in the past few hours is being propelled along by the smooth muscles of your digestive tract at about 2 mph. The planet beneath you rotates at more than 1,000 mph, speeding around a star at approximately 66,000 mph in a galaxy that is moving at more than 1 million mph through a universe that is continually expanding into the unknown. Likewise, at the quantum level, every particle in existence is appearing and disappearing in a dynamic state of vibrational existence we are only beginning to comprehend, all of it improbably held together in a balanced polarity of push-and-pull forces that allows you to hold this book and read its contents while sipping hot coffee from an open mug without scalding yourself or losing your place on the page. But the reality is that absolutely none of it is stationary at any time. It only *feels* that way. The universe and all matter contained within are in a highly organized state of fractal motion that is continually expanding through space and time.

The cosmic scale of this perpetual motion is imperceptible as you sit reading these pages, because Newton's laws (mostly the third) dictate that you can't experience the movement of a larger mass when you're connected to that mass and lack a fixed frame of reference—basically you don't know you're flying through space at a million miles an hour because you can't roll down your galactic passenger window and see a cosmic Burgerville disappearing in the sideview mirror. Of course, you also can't detect the microscopic bits of you, this book, or your beverage, which are all vibrating intensely with atomic energy, because they're moving on a scale too small to detect without highly specialized equipment. But, rest assured, perpetual motion is the inherent nature of all things—most importantly, your body. In fact, the human body is a unique biological organism that has evolved specifically to harness power from a universe in constant motion where gravity is king.

And this is where Newtonian physics begins to fail us as a model for understanding human movement.

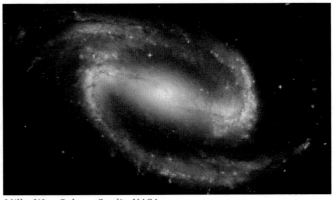

Milky Way Galaxy. Credit: NASA.

For as long as we've studied the science of athletic performance, we've largely looked at it through the lens of Newton's three laws of classical mechanics—where bodies are made of component parts with levered systems that have fulcrums and pivot points, and joints operate on a single plane of motion. As a result, anatomy textbooks have primarily dissected muscles to reveal the sagittal plane. And we have established the concept of "link action," where one bone remains still while the adjacent bone is articulated by muscle groups that shorten via concentric force, creating movement. And while this model is not wrong, it's only part of the equation. And it's only accurate if we put the body in a very restricted, artificial position. The reality is that when your body is in motion through space and time, it's doing multiple things at the same time on all three planes. Both the anchor bone and the action bone of a link action sequence are moving, as are many of the other bones and tissues around it. Multiple systems are simultaneously coordinating to harness power and momentum from the environment, so your body can channel force through a medium dominated by gravity in motion. While trainers and coaches have long conceptualized the human body as component parts that combine to create a highly refined machine, the reality is that human movement comes from the synchronized coordination of a symphony of systems all humming together in concert through time. Focusing on any one system too much inevitably compromises the others and weakens the whole. Our bodies are self-regenerating organisms that function more like plants than machines. And this requires a more natural, whole-system approach to understanding athletic performance than we have traditionally used.

The thing about Newton's laws of classical mechanics is that they are remarkably accurate for designing buildings, creating factories, assembling rockets, and launching them into orbit around other planets. But the human body operates according to *biological* laws. And biological laws are fundamentally different from mechanical laws. One of the key differences is that human bodies self-assemble using a chemically responsive process that continually adapts to its environment[1]. We are not machines assembled in a factory from boxes of component parts with different labels. And this is a crucial distinction. Because the fundamental drivers of biology are variability, resiliency, and *movement*—cellular movement, system movement, and organism movement. Without movement along these vectors, a biological organism will atrophy and die. The human body has adapted to move in a world that is itself in a state of constant motion and variability. This requires a combination of both stability and flexibility. And science is showing us that this balance of opposing forces is primarily enabled by the body's fascia system: the collagen and fluid-based matrix of elastic connective tissues surrounding your muscles and organs and suspending the structural framework of your bones together in a state of balanced tension like a tensegrity model[2].

What is a tensegrity model? I'm glad you asked. Grab your mug and lean in.

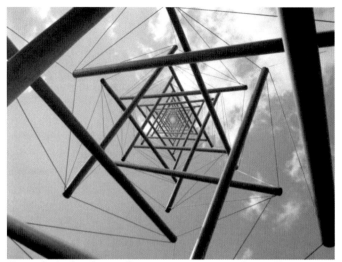

Kenneth Snelson's Needle Tower II is an 18-foot tall tensegrity sculpture at the Kroller-Muller Museum in the Netherlands.

Tensegrity (tension + integrity) is an architectural model that allows you to create stable but adaptable structures using a highly refined balance of tension and compression. In this model, solid struts are suspended without touching each other, floating in a state of equalized tension created by a network of pretensioned cables or bands. Originally coined by Buckminster Fuller as a structural term in the '60s, the concept was later extended to apply to biological systems by Dr. Stephen Levin, who dubbed the term, "biotensegrity[3]." In biology, bones provide the struts of a tensegrity system by constantly pushing out, while muscles and connective tissues provide the elastic center-seeking pulling force. In this model, the bones never really touch, and the body is an interconnected lever-less organism that adjusts to varying amounts of force and movement by distributing stress across the entire system. Tensegrity has become the foundation for a wide range of structure-based physical therapies, including yoga and Rolfing, as well as mechanical deep-tissue manipulations such as foam rolling and Active Release Technique (ART™). Tensegrity has even been applied by Harvard researcher, Donald Ingber, to explain cellular structures and functions in molecular biology[4]. Geometric patterns found in nature, including the DNA helix, can be accurately described as tension/compression systems that self-assemble in a way that efficiently uses the least amount of material necessary to create maximum structural resilience. This concept is important because it runs contrary to our traditional, compartmentalized Newtonian model for how bodies work. We are not Lego® people made of attached component parts. We are highly integrated, electrically activated, movement-enabled bio-structures that are held together in a state of stable yet flexible tension that is largely enabled by our body's viscoelastic fascia system.

If the phrase "fascia system" gives you pause or prompts you to think of its better-known (and frequently injured) component parts—like ligaments and tendons—it's not an accident. As anatomy expert and creator of Anatomy Trains®, Thomas Myers, explains: "Fascia is the Cinderella of body tissues, anatomically misunderstood and systematically ignored." This is because the fascia system—which runs throughout your entire body, head to toe, supporting every organ, muscle, and bone in you[5]—is a single interconnected web of collagen and pressurized fluid that virtually disappears when the human body is dissected. It's essentially a sealed hydraulic system that functions only when you're alive. It is routinely just removed and discarded as part of the dissection process.

Modern imaging technologies, like ultrasound, are just now allowing us to see this system as it exists in the living body. In fact, after more than 500 years of anatomical study, we still don't have a single comprehensive image of the fascia system, like we do of the circulatory and musculoskeletal systems. Due to this elusive invisibility, and the fact that human anatomy has long been viewed through a Newtonian lens of individualized parts, the body's fascia network has not traditionally been recognized as a single cohesive system, and its role in athletic performance has been greatly underestimated.

"In dissection, fascia is literally a greasy mess that's everywhere—what you see in textbooks has had all the fascia cleaned off—and its structure is so variable between different people that its physical architecture is hard to delineate," says Myers.

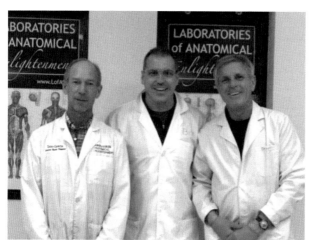

Bill Parisi (C) with master dissectionist Todd Garcia (L) and Tom Myers (R) at the Anatomy Trains Human Dissection Course in Boulder, Colorado.

While fascia may not have interested science much in the past few hundred years, your brain sure wants to know a lot about it. In fact, according to current research, the fascia system contains about six times more sensory nerve endings than muscle, making it essentially a body-wide sensory organ[6].

It also has tremendous tensile properties that serve to stabilize the body, distribute force, and amplify motion. And, as Davis's Law states, it continually remodels itself based on stress, load, pressure, and vibration[7]. This means that fascia is one of your body's most trainable systems. In fact, you are born with your entire fascia system intact, and you spend every minute of your life training it—whether you're aware of it or not—because it's always rebuilding itself in response to the stress placed on it by your movement (or lack thereof), your diet, and your daily habits. Every cell in your body is connected to the suspension network of this one system. Think of your fascia system as the space-organizing substructure that connects everything in you and holds it in place, providing a flexible platform for stability in a continually moving world.

Or, to put it another way, if a billionaire entrepreneur provided you with the resources necessary to develop an artificial human, you would have basically two routes: Build a Newtonian robot—like C-3PO or the DARPA Dog—assembled out of component parts, including levers, pivot points, and hydraulic systems. Or go the bio route and create a self-organizing, humanoid—more akin to the replicants of Blade Runner or the residents of Westworld—that can move with the same grace, precision, and lethality as actual humans. Of course, creating an android capable of moving with the power and fluidity of a professional athlete would be magnitudes of difficulty more complex using current technology. It would first necessitate the development of an electrically active soft tissue with high tensile-strength that can retain shape under uneven loads, sudden stress, and rapid movements. You would essentially need to start by developing an artificial fascia system. PS: This is currently in development[8].

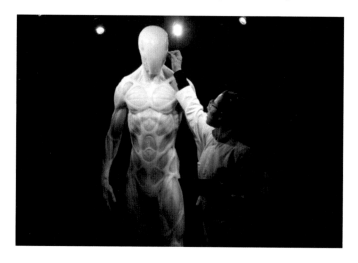

Like many athletes and trainers, I've been intuitively aware of the importance of connective tissue in athletic performance since my early career. I've found that different types of athletes can be successfully categorized into different animal classes based on their body type and sport. Take, for example, the cheetah. Cheetahs are lean, super-fast, and sparse on muscle. Athletes in the cheetah category often include wide receivers and defensive backs. Cheetah athletes have low body fat and long, powerful, spring-like tendons with lots of elasticity. Athletes in the rhino category have more muscle bulk and brute strength but are also fast and explosive.

Think of fullbacks, tight ends, and LeBron James. Giraffes are long and tall but also fast and powerful. Athletes in the giraffe category include centers and forwards in basketball. These kinds of animal classifications have helped me develop highly personalized training programs and recovery times for each type of athlete I've worked with throughout my career. But only recently have I had the paradigm shift that whole-system, fascia-focused training deserves, in large part, because it keeps coming up in different ways from different studies and experts who are all at the top of their field.

As Exhibit A, I offer you the humble kangaroo.

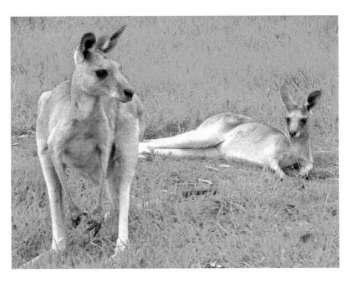

While kangaroos possess the same kind of marsupial muscle tissues as koala bears, they have the remarkable ability to jump more than 40 feet at a time in rapid sequence when being pursued by whatever it is that eats kangaroos (or if there's a really good kangaroo party going down). Intrigued by the biological improbability, researchers discovered that this extraordinary superpower for generating force is attributed to the fact that kangaroos have hyper-developed tendons in their hind legs that give them an unparalleled ability to store and release kinetic energy using an elastic dynamic called the "catapult effect.[9]" In this dynamic, the surrounding muscles pre-contract to stretch the attached connective tissues—loading them like a stretched rubber band—then quickly release this stored elastic energy with an explosive pulse of force. Gazelles have this feature too. And recent ultrasound imaging has allowed us to see that humans are unique among bipeds, because we are the only two-legged species on the planet that also has this type of elastic kinetic storage system[10]. But our capacity for elastic energy storage and recoil has so far remained relatively under-appreciated and untrained.

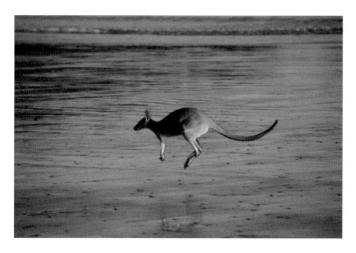

Likewise, a University of Tokyo study[11] of fascia and connective tissues, analyzing ultrasound data generated by athletes using a lying leg-lift machine to simulate jumping, revealed that elastic connective tissues—not muscles—are responsible for most of the power generation in explosive actions like jumping and running. The data showed that muscle fibers work almost isometrically and leave the task of storing and releasing elastic energy to the tendons. This allows muscles to pulse and relax as necessary to maintain maximum efficiency and optimize power in quick repetitive cycles.

Additionally, measurements of calf lengthening during running have shown that much of the length required for dorsiflexion comes from the elastic stretching of fascia tissue, while the muscles contract isometrically[12].

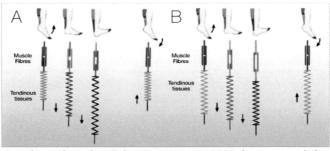

A study conducted at Tokyo University in 2002 demonstrated that the pulsing elastic properties of fascia tissue are more responsible for power generation in running than muscle.

This data contradicts previous perceptions that tendons are simply non-elastic plastic wrap, and that muscles lengthen and shorten during cyclic running motions. This was a huge realization for me. For years, trainers have fixated on increasing power by making athletes stronger—focusing on specific muscle groups or body parts—without appreciating the significance of the underlying fascia system and how it works to harness, distribute, and amplify force across the body.

Michol Dalcourt, Director of the Institute of Motion and creator of the ViPR PRO™ loaded-movement training tool[13], discovered this early in his career while training hockey players at the University of Alberta.

"My viewpoint at the time was strongly rooted in the notion that we are made up of constituent parts," says Dalcourt. "I thought training these parts one by one was the most important factor for success. For three years I trained hockey players to develop their speed, strength, and agility in a 14-week off-season training program. Then, every season, I would ask the scouts how my players were doing."

For three years, the answer never changed: "They need to improve their strength on the puck."

Dalcourt found this odd, because strength was exactly what he thought he was training for. This prompted him to ask the obvious follow-up: "Who's beating my players to the puck?"

The inevitable answer was always, "The farm kids."

"Everyone in the sport knew the toughest players were the farm kids," says Dalcourt. "But it made little sense on the surface. They didn't train with weights in a gym; they didn't periodize training stress. They would rarely overload a muscle or perform the same motion repeatedly to get stronger. While the gym kids often looked bigger and stronger, these farm kids were truly *functional*. Everything they did was performed with varying loads, in all three planes, at various speeds, and with various ranges of motion.

They simply called it 'doing chores'—moving farm equipment, shoveling, lifting things, squatting, crouching, rotating, lunging, pushing, pulling, etc. There was always a task-based objective, and their bodies got the job done as efficiently as possible. Isolation training doesn't exist on the farm, because it's too inefficient. The body is naturally designed to spread forces and stress out into the system, through each joint and tissue in the body. The more effectively that is accomplished, the less injury will plague the system. I found that as soon as I adopted similar strategies in my training, my players became stronger, quicker, and more agile, with far less incidence of injury."

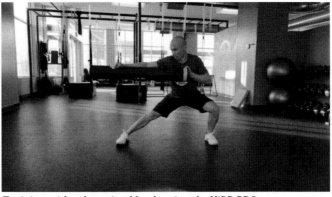

Training with submaximal loads using the ViPR PRO.

I experienced one of my own *"aha!"* moments while traveling around the country with my teenage son, Will, who was playing alongside many of the country's top youth basketball players in the Nike-sponsored AAU Tournament. I was amazed at the natural ability many of these 15- and 16-year-old city kids had to cross the floor in five or six strides, play above the rim, and dunk at will.

These were lean, lanky teenagers without a lot of muscle. But their explosive athleticism was tremendous. One of the secrets to my success has long been that whenever I see an exceptional athlete, I make a point of pulling them aside and asking them about their training techniques and who their coaches are. When I asked these kids what they did for training, the universal answer was always that they just played basketball. And that's when I realized: These kids were the natural result of fascia training!

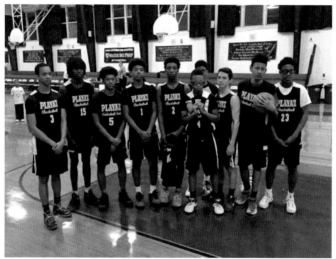

Who wants to play: Which kid's name is Parisi?!

As a dynamically responsive system, your fascia tissue continually remodels itself based on the things you do every day. These kids played basketball. A *lot* of basketball—for hours on end, day after day— most of them without ever setting foot in a weight room.

And their fascia systems developed accordingly, adapting over time in response to the rhythmic bouncing and explosive dynamics of the game, to give them kangaroo-like abilities for running, jumping, and rapidly changing directions. While these young athletes will obviously need an individually tailored amount of traditional weightlifting and eccentric loading as part of a balanced training program to improve their strength and injury resilience, focusing too much on building their muscles to increase power will actually end up slowing them down, reducing their jump height, impairing their proprioception, and increasing their chance of injury. I've seen it happen to athletes in every sport more times than I can count. The reality is that optimizing an athlete's inherent genetic potential requires a whole-system approach that maximizes the biomechanical advantages of their connective tissues in balance with their musculoskeletal, nervous, and cardiovascular systems.

And this led me to the question: How do we enhance the inherent biological advantages of an athlete's fascia system while also incorporating everything else we've learned about strength conditioning and neural control to create a safer, more effective approach to training?

So, of course ... I set out on a nationwide quest to ask the experts.

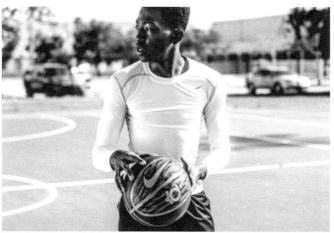

Basketball naturally amplifies elastic fascia training by demanding rapid changes in direction with explosive movements and highly variable, sub-maximal loads in a wide range of vectors.

Bill Parisi / Johnathon Allen

The Fascia System: A New Understanding

IF WE'RE GOING TO DEVELOP a better approach to speed and power training that acknowledges fascia's significant role in performance and injury prevention, it's critical we have a better understanding of what it is and how it works. Given that we're only just now beginning to recognize it as a singular system, this is no small task. The International Fascial Research Congress[14]—which convened in Berlin for the fifth time ever in November, 2018—is still defining the exact parameters of its features and properties. And the terminology surrounding it continues to be in flux, as different professionals in the field still refer to it by different, often interchangeable, names including: "the fascial system," the "extra cellular matrix (ECM)," and "the myofascial web," among others. For the purposes of this book, I've chosen to refer to it simply as "the fascia system." Since paradigm shifts are hard enough. But you will hear many of the experts we interview along the way refer to it using an array of terms.

This includes one of the world's preeminent authorities on the subject, Thomas Myers, creator of Anatomy Trains, a detailed map of the connected lines of force transmission (or "Trains") through the body's myofascial web. As a self-described "consumer of research," bodywork instructor, and seeker of knowledge, Thomas has been traveling the globe since the mid-'70s studying under top minds (including Buckminster Fuller and Ida Rolf), performing instructional anatomical dissections, and conducting courses on how to use the Anatomy Trains, all in the pursuit of developing a more complete understanding of how the fascia system works. Driving up the coast from Portland, Maine, to interview him, it occurs to me the man has probably forgotten more about the subject than I will ever know.

"We are accustomed to identifying individual structures within the fascial web—like the plantar fascia, the Achilles tendon, the iliotibial band, thoracolumbar aponeurosis, nuchal ligament, and so on—but these are just labels for zip codes within the singular fascial web," says Myers, as he tacks his sailboat in a stiff wind through the sunlit waters off the coast of the Anatomy Trains headquarters in Walpole, Maine.

"We can talk about the Atlantic, the Pacific, and the Mediterranean oceans, but there is really only *one* interconnected ocean in the world. Fascia is the same. If it could be magically extracted as a whole, your fascial web would outline all the detailed shapes of your body, inside and out. It would be one intricate net with muscles squirming in it like swimming fish. Every organ and cell is embedded within this unitary sea of a fascial net. Understanding this is important, because we are so strongly inclined to identify individual anatomical structures by saying things like, 'Oh, you tore your biceps,' forgetting that the word *biceps* is just a construct, because our traditional scientific nomenclature creates a false impression."

That Thomas frequently uses nautical metaphors to describe the fascia system is no accident. Watching him casually navigate his 35-foot Bristol yawl through the bobbing maze of lobster buoys floating in the bay that has been in his family for generations, it's clear his first passion is sailing.

His parents took him along on sailing trips as an infant, and he's been practicing the craft since he was old enough to hold a rope. When the opportunity strikes, he sails away from the Anatomy Trains headquarters for weeks at a time, following the winds and currents around the secluded islands of Acadia.

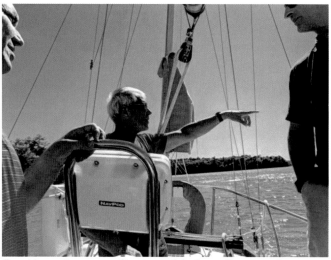

Tom Myers gives us a sailing tour of the bay adjacent to the Anatomy Trains headquarters in Walpole, Maine. Credit: Johnathon Allen.

"Sailing has probably taught me more about the fascial system than anything else," says Myers.

It makes sense. The fascia system *is* mostly water (and collagen) under hydraulic pressure, after all. And these are newly charted waters that quickly get deep when you dive into them, so, metaphors are handy. Which is why I'm going to do my best to outline the basic principles of fascia training as they relate to athletic performance while trying to keep things clear and usable for the average person.

If I get in over my head, I'll ask Thomas to throw me a lifeline. As a 5'10" Italian from Jersey, getting in over my head is sort of a thing I do. That said, if you want to understand the deeper science for yourself, I encourage you to reference the attributions, endnotes, and experts cited in this book. Grab the ball and run with it! There's a lot to know, and new information is coming out every day.

So, what exactly *is* fascia tissue?

Well, the short answer is that fascia is a "colloid," which is a mix of collagen fibers suspended in liquid gels. This makes it *both* a fiber and a fluid and gives fascia the viscoelastic properties of a non-Newtonian fluid when under load. This means that fascia has a diverse range of structural features that are based on the length, shape, and density of the collagen fibers, and the viscosity of the gels they mix with. Key features of fascia tissue include: viscosity (the ability of tissues to slide against each other), elasticity (the ability of tissue to store and release kinetic energy), and plasticity (the ability of tissue to resist distortion and to reshape itself along lines of stress).

There are also different types of fascia tissue that are primarily differentiated by which layer they are on. "Superficial fascia" is the loose layer directly beneath your skin that allows you to pick your skin up off your body. Its viscoelastic properties buffer your skin from the muscles to allow for a smooth sliding action between them, while also allowing your skin to return to its normal tension level after you do things like fall asleep in a beach chair for two hours or lose weight. Similar loose fascia also surrounds the organs, glands, nerve bundles, and other interstitial spaces in your body, playing a significant role in thermoregulation, circulation, insulation, and lymphatic flow.

"Deep fascia" is the thick, highly fibrous internal bodysuit that includes pockets (epimysium) surrounding each individual muscle, and broad, flat sheaths (aponeuroses) that cover muscle groups, as well as connective joint tissues like tendons and ligaments. "Deep fascia" is the layer where myofascial force transmission happens[15]. Its dense collagen fibers are similar to a powerlifter's elastic bodysuit or an NBA player's shooting sleeve—but on the *inside*—suspending your muscles in a state of tension that allows them to operate. Research has shown that muscles transmit up to 40 percent of their contraction force into adjacent muscles—including antagonistic muscles that are co-stiffened to increase resistance—via deep fascial connections[16]. This means force transmission through these myofascial linkages, or "trains," in your body is much greater than we've traditionally assumed.

The basic components of fascia tissue are created by cells (mostly fibroblasts) that extrude through the Extra Cellular Matrix (ECM). The ECM provides a fluid-based scaffolding for everything in your body and enables mechanical signaling between cells and systems. Aside from the collagen and elastin fibers, the fluid part of ECM is called "ground substance," which is a clear, watery gel that varies in viscoelasticity depending on the number of fibers and amount of water and other chemicals present. The synovial fluid in your joints is essentially a gel mixed with a lot of water, while the cartilage on the ends of your bones is made of a similar gel with very little water. But my favorite character in the fascia universe is the fibroblast. Fibroblast cells are the biomechanical architects of the system, producing fibers in the ECM like little cellular spiders spinning out a double-lattice web of collagen and other chemicals along the directional lines of stress occurring within the matrix. They also secrete collagenase, which is an enzyme that eats collagen in areas where it's no longer needed, or where it's so old that it's fraying—removing and rebuilding fibers as they go. The best part is that these little dudes detect ongoing pressure and vibration signals coming into the ECM and respond on a localized supply-and-demand basis. This has tremendous implications from a training standpoint.

"You have literally millions of these little fibroblasts crawling around your body leaving a trail of slime behind them. But it's your movement that organizes that slime," says Myers. "The fibroblast can't do anything but leave it behind. It doesn't build bone. It doesn't build cartilage. Forces build those things. So, what happens after this latticework comes out of the fibroblast is entirely dependent on the forces you put into the body. Load makes the cell go there by creating an ionic flow in the tissue that these cells are listening to. So, when you put load on the tissue, those cells migrate there and lay down traffic. Then you come along and organize it with your movement and loading—hopefully in a positive way."

This means that when you train fascia tissue consciously and correctly over time, you can develop robust strands of long collagen fibers with high tensile strength that have tremendous resilience and elastic storage capabilities. The flipside is that injuries, surgeries, lack of activity, improper form, and excessive repetitive motions can all weaken and damage fascia tissue, leading to chronic injuries, postural imbalances, tissue binding, weak joints, and other complications.

"Carved in large letters over the gate are the words: *THE BODY RESPONDS TO DEMAND*," says Myers, echoing Wolff's Law[17].

"When you generate force through the body, it gets handled by joints, muscles, skeleton, and fascia. If you don't put the demand on the body to make connections among these various tissues, they won't develop. The problem with a lot of the power and speed training techniques I've seen is that they focus on building the muscle before the fascia. The fascia is a Saint Bernard. It's got the brandy, but it walks more slowly up the mountain. That's why the onramp for traditional disciplines like martial arts and yoga is slower than in western training, because they intuitively understood that injury is likely to happen three or four months into training, if you don't build a resilient fascia foundation first."

Research also shows that leveraging the elastic fascial recoil energy in your tendons during explosive movements amplifies the motion while reducing the demand on your muscles—which makes movements easier, more controllable, and more efficient. But as Myers points out, building up this elasticity is a matter of putting demand on the tissues. This means that a foundational element of fascia training is to start out doing movements slowly with proper form and then increasing speed and load as the tissue and nervous system mature and adapt. While significant muscle development can be achieved in a matter of weeks and months, it can take six months to two years to build up balanced body-wide fascia elasticity.

"Fascial elasticity is important, because most tearing injuries occur when connective tissue is stretched faster than it can respond. This is one reason why soft tissue injuries are really common three or four months into a new training regime. The muscles typically develop much faster than fascial elasticity, and the greater the imbalance between the two, the higher the chance for injury," says Myers.

The thing about fascial elasticity is that elastic energy is stored and released by fascia very quickly, in less than 1.2 seconds[18]. If a force lasts longer than that, the plasticity properties of fascia will adjust to accommodate to the load and cause it to stretch in much the same way a plastic bag will deform under the stress of your groceries. This means that training for improved elasticity requires short, cyclic, quickly repeated motions, like bouncing, jumping rope, or running on the balls of your feet (as opposed to slower-contraction cycles, like bicycling or rowing). This isn't to say that slow contractions don't train fascia, because *everything you do trains fascia tissue.* It's just that those movements don't develop *fascial elasticity.* They develop other features. Traditional loading with weights can improve fiber thickness and strengthen ligament and tendon connections with surrounding muscle tissues, while stretching and yoga can lengthen fibers to improve fluid flow. But recovery and remodeling take time, and fascia is weaker as it rebuilds, which means, for example, that you don't want to do intense stretching followed by a day of heavy lifting.

"When you put fascia tissue under load, it squeezes water out of the tendon like a sponge, until the load is released, and the water is sucked back in. The more hydrated the tissue, the less likely you are to injure it. But when you're talking about training for elasticity, the goal is to very quickly squeeze water out of the tendons just long enough for the double lattice to arrange itself and set into the molecular structure. Then you let the tension go. Thanks to that new lattice structure, the tendon won't suck as much water back in, and the tissue will become less soggy and more elastic over time," says Myers.

Conversely, properly prescribed isotonic weightlifting will help develop other properties that can improve the structural integrity of tendons, ligaments, and connective tissues to help keep joints safe under the tremendous speeds, reaction times, and rotational forces experienced by professional athletes.

"When you do a loaded bench press or squat, you're squeezing water out of the matrix of those tissues for the moment that you're doing the exercise—the time under tension. The thickness, complexity, and resilience of the fibers will be determined by that time under tension.

"So, the tendons are going to get thicker and stronger and have more hydroxyl bonds, but those steady loads aren't going to create more elasticity. It's really a matter of what you're training for. The important part is that you need to train the fascial tissue before you get into things like speed or power training, so that everything is balanced. In sailing for example, I need all my guy wires, shrouds, and stays to have about the same amount of tension or I'm going to bust my boat in high winds. Athletes competing in high performance sports are all under high winds in that analogy. So, regardless of what you're training for, you need some form of pretraining and conditioning that helps you get all the myofascial units involved to be about the same level of tone.

Isolated areas of extra-high tone or low tone predispose an athlete to injury, but when you have an even tone across the body, you'll have the most injury resilience," says Myers.

And this brings us back to the importance of personalized coaching and an individualized approach to training. Every athlete/animal, sport, and situation is unique. That's why it's critical to have the most complete, up-to-date toolset possible for assessing each individual and goal.

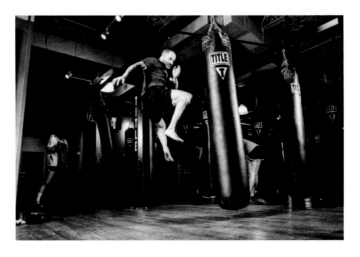

One thing every sport comes down to—whether it involves running, jumping, kicking, hitting, or throwing—is the ability to generate a lot of force very fast. Rapid force generation is also the foundation for most martial arts disciplines. It takes years of training and practice to develop blackbelt levels of power production. But as fighters progress from beginners to blackbelts, they don't typically add a lot of muscle girth. They get better at recruiting muscular units, developing more motor-engrams, and channeling more force.

Obviously, the fascia system plays a role in all of this. So, I asked Thomas, "How does the fascia system contribute to a professional fighter's ability to generate force?"

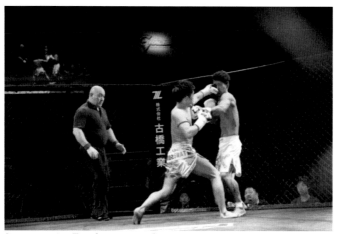

Interoceptive Totality to your face! Source: PXHere

"I've never put this into a term before, but I would call it: *Interoceptive Totality.* Basically, they've learned to channel force using their entire body rather than just bits and pieces. There are limitations to training when you're just working bits and pieces. You can focus on training individual muscles, and it feels good. But when you come at something with speed and force, your entire body is involved. When you start the pre-load cycle to drop into a movement before you explode, your brain is checking out every tissue you're dropping into, particularly the joints, probing to see: Is my ankle ready for this; is my foot ready; is my knee ready; are my hips ready; is my back ready? If it doesn't check out, you will abort or modify things in a serious way. But if it all checks out then, *BOOM,* you will explode.

"It's a combination of proprioception and interoception—how you feel about what you sense in your body. To master it, you want to train progressively, starting with slow whole-body movements that allow you to recruit the most neuromuscular units during the movement and stimulate the most tissues. Then, over time, you can ramp up your speed and power to achieve greater levels of force with lower risk of injury."

The idea is that when you start out training slowly with good form, you allow the entire fabric of all of the involved systems to engage in the action. This added dimension of connectivity will then be recruited for increased force production, stability, and speed.

"I use the practice of moving slowly with my clients, to make sure they're including all the parts that they don't take the time to think about when they're moving fast. Or to put it another way: Just because you can do something fast, doesn't mean you can do it slowly," says Myers.

Then I watched as Thomas demonstrated his own Interoceptive Totality by gracefully guiding his 35-foot sailboat loaded with five adult males to a smooth, gentle stop alongside his dock like a falcon effortlessly landing on a branch. It took me a moment to realize I'd never seen anyone dock a boat entirely under sail like that, without a motor. And then I remembered we were in the presence of a master, a man at the center of his domain, where wind, sail, and sinew all come together in a seamless symmetry of precision, a symphony of systems in perfect tune with the elements.

And then we went to lunch.

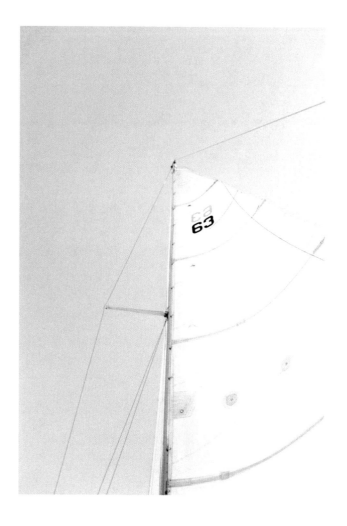

Whole-System Training: Isokinetic Resistance

I CAN PRACTICALLY HEAR YOU on the other side of the page right now thinking, "OK, Bill ... that's all fine and good, and everybody loves a fun road trip story about sailing and kangaroos, but how do we actually apply this information to improve athletic performance and reduce injury?" That's why I invited physicist and inventor, Dave Schmidt, developer of Optimal Human Motion (OHM™) Dynamics—a new isokinetic "reactive resistance" modality—to join me for lunch at a dockside restaurant in Portland, Maine, to chat about that subject after meeting with Thomas. Also, after seeing all of those floating buoys in the bay, I had a sudden craving for fresh lobster salad.

I originally met Dave in 2017 while I was a speaker at the national PerformBetter Summit series. Chris Poirier, manager of PerformBetter—one of the biggest athletic performance equipment distributors in the world—tipped me to Dave and his newly developed isokinetic platform, because it was based on the same whole-body training principles we use at the Parisi Speed School. Dave describes his modality as advancing previous forms of isokinetic technology with a new form of accommodating resistance that allows you to exert maximum force in any direction, on any plane of motion, and it will provide a fluid amount of responsive resistance. Basically, the harder and faster you push, the more resistance you get back. When you stop, it stops. This means you can maximize force output by training through your entire range of motion, allowing you to increase motor unit recruitment and connective tissue engagement throughout the entire sequence. The very first time I tried Dave's equipment, I knew it was a game changer. Somehow, this crazy smart inventor from Connecticut with a background in physics and no formal sports training had evolved a new modality for exercise, in his garage, out of pure curiosity and a desire to create something that didn't exist: a *fun* piece of performance training equipment that simulates real-world physics.

After meeting him, I persuaded Dave to let us keep two of his early beta units at our training facility in Fair Lawn for in-house testing and research. After testing his equipment for most of a year, we've seen tremendous results with athletes at the highest levels of competition. Just to clarify, I'm not trying to sell you Dave's equipment. But I've been so impressed with how well it works, I wanted to talk to him about why.

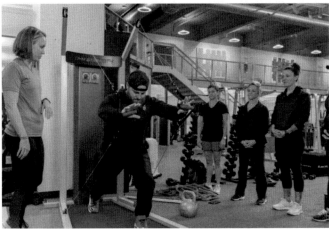

Debuting an OHM Strength machine at the Chelsea Piers Fitness Center in New York. Credit: Jonathan Cunningham.

A notable example is one of our Parisi Speed School coaches—22-year-old George Alexandris. George recently started training to get back into collegiate track and field, competing for the Montclair State Red Hawks, after taking two years off to focus on becoming a Parisi Performance Coach. Coming back to his training regime, he decided to reduce the amount of traditional weightlifting he'd been doing and replace it with a more whole-body, fascia-based approach using Dave's test equipment at our facility, in conjunction with medicine ball and other natural resistance techniques. His first big payoff came when he won the 2018 NCAA Division III Outdoor Track and Field Championships in the long jump, with a distance of 26 feet—breaking the competition's 44-year-old record.

Weeks later, he posted an Instagram video of himself running 26 miles per hour on Fair Lawn's high-speed treadmill—and holding that speed for five seconds[19]. It was insane! He got over three million views in less than two days. And while I understood why he was getting these kinds of results, I wanted to get Dave's perspective on how his new technology fits into all of this.

But before we get to that, I need to bring you up to speed on a little historical context. So, hop in the passenger seat of my time-travelling DeLorean, and we'll take a quick flashback to the '80s, as we drive down the Maine Turnpike in search of fresh lobster salad and an oceanside deck with a view. A key thing to keep in mind here is that, while advanced new technologies are emerging that allow us to better understand—and train—our fascia tissue and other systems, many of these approaches aren't new. It's our understanding of why and how they work that has changed.

I've been successfully using whole-system, three-dimensional training methods my entire life. It's what the Parisi Speed School is built on. And our results over the past two-plus decades prove their effectiveness. But only recently have I really begun to understand the science behind *why*. So, let's roll the cosmic odometer back to the mid-'80s—when Back to the Future actually came out—and cue the fluorescent-lit interior of a high school gym in northern New Jersey, crowded with old-school Universal gym equipment and testosterone-fueled teenage jocks. I'm a thick, undersized, mildly athletic teenager interested in throwing the javelin—a sport that math says I should be underwhelming at, even on a good day. Traditional weight training was what you did back then to develop power. So, I did all the standard exercises: squats, bench presses, deadlifts. I put on a little size; I got a little stronger; I got a little faster. But somewhere in my junior year, our little high school gym got a brand-new piece of equipment called "the Leaper."

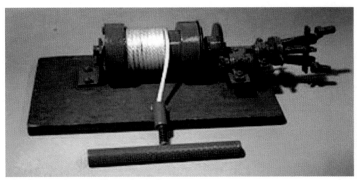

The first isokinetic "home gym."

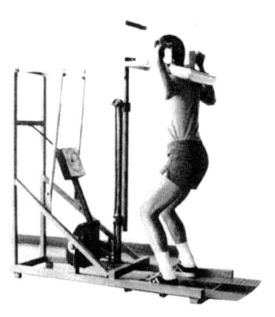

Glen Henson created The Leaper in 1974, revolutionizing the fitness industry.

It was an isokinetic exercise machine with a chain and a shoulder harness that allowed you to do a squat motion while pushing up with 100 percent effort, so you could keep maxing out your efforts all the way through a full range of motion. It was explosive, dynamic, and totally different from lifting weights—which is a closed kinetic chain movement where you slow down at the end of each rep to control the momentum and gravity of the weight. My approach with the Leaper was to do 10 to 20 reps per set, for multiple sets, as hard as I could go. It would really fatigue me, but it wouldn't make me sore the next day.

It maximized my training efforts by allowing me to squeeze every ounce of effort out of myself every time. I didn't think much of it back then, other than that it was a great workout.

But then I noticed after about six weeks or so of doing it, I was jumping and grabbing the basketball rim and smoking the running backs in gym class sprints even though I had the body of a linebacker. Training on that machine did *something* to me I didn't entirely understand, but I knew it worked. It was the first piece of a puzzle I'm just now beginning to see come together through new advancements in technology and research.

When I got to Iona College, I was excited to see they also had one of these isokinetic machines, but it was designed for training the upper body. It was mostly being used by the swim team. So I modified it a little to simulate a javelin throw, allowing me to work through the same range of motion against a steady form of resistance. This ended up being a huge contributor to my athletic success. Again, short stocky Italians aren't genetically predisposed to throwing aluminum spears. We excel more in the punching, cooking, talking shit, watching Rocky, and driving fast on summer nights with the windows down listening to Bruce Springsteen categories. Great javelin throwers are typically tall, lean, eastern Europeans and Norwegians. Yet, using a combination of isokinetic training, 10,000-plus med ball throws every off-season, and other three-dimensional whole-body techniques, I rose to the top of the collegiate competitive field and got my education paid for by becoming one of the best NCAA Division I javelin throwers in the nation and the all-time record holder at Iona College.

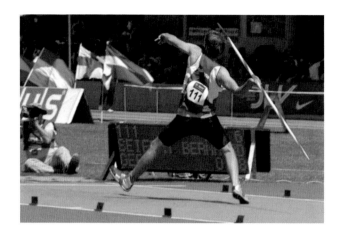

And that's when I realized that being good at throwing is one of the most complete forms of athleticism you can have. To be a great thrower, you need a powerful lower body and a stiff, super-strong core, because you're generating all of the force from your lower body—channeling it from your feet and legs all the way through your trunk, torso, shoulder, arm, elbow, wrist, and fingers. You need to transfer power through your entire body at the most fundamental levels. And these principles apply to all types of sports and skills—whether it's football, basketball, hockey, jiu jitsu, or golf. They're all about the transfer of energy and power, either vertically into the ground, horizontally from one foot to the other, or propulsively into another object. The discoveries I made in the process of learning to throw a javelin better apply to every athlete. But they're also as old as time. Or at least as old as Neanderthals throwing rocks.

The cool part is that now we live in the 21st century, and our technology and training tools are finally catching up to how our bodies actually work.

This is thanks in no small part to inventors like Dave Schmidt who have a never-ending obsession with gaining a better understanding of how the universe works and a late-night habit of creating things that don't already exist.

"I studied physics, not physiology," says Dave. "So I'm coming at some of these ideas as a complete outsider, which has turned out to be very valuable, because I don't have the blinders on that a conventional education might have given me. This means I'm able to think outside the box, explore my own ideas, and come up with new approaches for making functional fitness equipment without being burdened by too much preexisting bias."

This from a guy who at 12 years old built a hang glider in his parents' garage so he could fly himself down the beach where his family lived. Now—still living on the shores of that same secluded bay with his wife and three kids—Dave continues making things in his garage, including a custom-designed rowing dory he uses for fitness, a ukulele, and a 55-foot waterslide his son has used to help catapult himself into being a competitive collegiate diver. To me, one of the most interesting things about Dave is that his new modality wasn't born out of a desire to revolutionize the fitness industry. It came out of the basic human desire for fun—which is not a term normally associated with athletic training equipment.

"My quest to build this kind of exercise equipment started with my experience using a NordicTrack cross-country ski machine. I love cross-country skiing because it allows me to glide through nature and produce power in a way that makes me feel like the perfect human. Yet when I got on this training machine, I had to learn something completely different.

And once I learned that something different—sure, I was able to NordicTrack, but it didn't give me the same euphoria I experienced when I was outside skiing in the snow. It was like riding a stationary bike—which I also dislike—because it feels sluggish and unnatural, like riding a bike when I'm sick with the flu. It doesn't maintain momentum. This is tied to the phenomenal way our bodies are proprioceptive in everything we do. That's when I started thinking about the forces we generate to propel ourselves through nature and how they differ from the kinds of equipment that we've traditionally worked out with in gyms."

I could tell Dave was about to put his physics hat on and things were going to get nerdy. Also, my lobster salad had just landed. So I picked up my fork and asked him to explain.

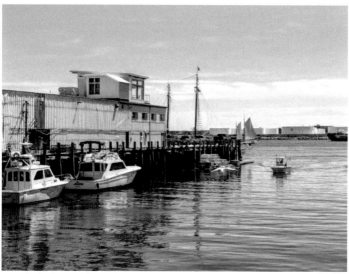

Lunch deck view from the Porthole restaurant, Portland, Maine.
Credit: Johnathon Allen.

"Fun was really the thing I was looking for. And this led me to wondering how we could replicate the experience of moving through nature *inside*. That's when I realized the importance of variable resistance in human movement—the ability to dictate what level of force we apply to generate power—particularly when we're in a propulsive mode. When you're moving through nature—whether you're rowing a boat, riding a bike, swimming, running, or whatever— you get to choose how hard you push at all points through the range of motion. Our ability to do that means we can load our bodies in the most optimal way for the task at hand while also reducing our risk of injury. When I was younger, the goal in a gym was always to push yourself to failure. They said, 'Choose enough weight so you can do 10 or 12 reps, but on your last rep, you want to be failing.' Of course, those first bunch of reps were fairly easy. I wasn't pushing as hard as I really could. But as I began to fatigue, it became harder and harder. Now, I know that for my joints to operate properly, my muscles need to be firing properly. And when my muscles start to fail, my joints begin to see significant loads. I'm putting greater compressive forces on the connective tissues in those joints. It makes all the sense in the world to me now that pushing to failure, especially under a fixed gravitational force, is a sure-fire way of inviting injury. When I go out rowing, I can pull as hard as I want on that very first stroke. I can put 100 percent of my effort into it. A thousand strokes later, I may still be putting in 100 percent effort, but the force I'm producing is much lower. By the time I get back to the beach after an hour-long row, I might be down to 70 percent of my original effort, but it doesn't matter. I'm never pushing myself to failure.

"I'm pushing myself optimally to produce the power I can produce. But let's stop for a moment and talk about how we define power."

See, I knew this was going to get nerdy. Also, this salad is delicious. Proceed.

"Power is the key to success for any athlete. To be able to optimize power, you want to work in a training environment where you're able to exercise the way your body naturally moves. In physics, we define power as *force times speed*. When you start moving faster and faster while pushing a heavy amount of force, you're not able to keep that force up, but your speed is gaining. If you look at the product of the two combined—force and speed—you can see the force drop, but as long as your speed is increasing, you may still be generating higher and higher power numbers. Just like when you ride a bike. You're looking for the perfect combination of cadence and force by shifting gears. When you find that perfect gear, it allows you to deliver the most power into the bike and go the fastest. That's when you're producing optimal power. It's a combination of force and speed. My thought process on the subject has evolved to focus on the difference between how we interact with gravity versus how we handle propulsion. In physics, the difference is very clear.

When something is a gravitational force, such as a weight or a heavy rock, it's defined by the gravitational constant of the Earth multiplied by the mass of the object. Those are both constants, which means the force you need to apply to counter that gravity is also a constant.

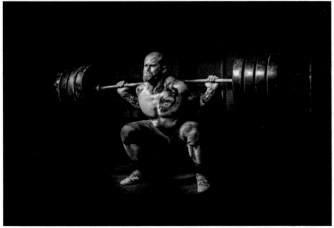

Gravitational force is a fixed constant. Source: PXHere.

"It's just math. And that constant is something our bodies subconsciously keep in mind when we're dealing with gravity. When you go to lift something heavy, your body gets in a very different position than when you're in a state of propulsion. When you push or pull against something, it's happening in a horizontal plane that's defined in physics as *force equals mass times acceleration.*

"So, the force you produce is really based on how quickly and how hard you accelerate something.

"If you and I are pushing against each other in a football game—your mass against my mass—the faster I accelerate as I push you, the greater the force is that I need to produce. The beauty in that exchange is that I can alter my force output and acceleration a million times throughout the motion—from the very beginning to the very end—and I do it seamlessly without even thinking about it.

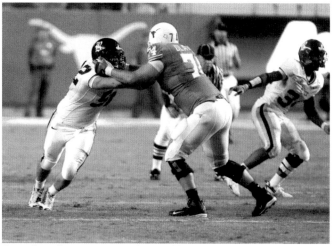

Propulsive force is constantly variable. Source: PXHere.

"The propulsive force you produce is tremendously variable, but, more importantly, it matches your physiology. When you're dealing with gravity, the force is dictated. It's already decided when you pick up an object how much force you will need to lift it, and at no time can you let up, or you're going to drop the object."

Allow me to put the nerd cap on for a moment. For a long time, I've felt very strongly that our industry puts too much emphasis on heavy weight training. And I've known that training with full body movements using isokinetic tools like the Leaper and functional training tools like the medicine ball are the keys to developing explosive power. But here's the big drumroll moment: After looking at the research data, I have come to believe that there are two secrets behind this approach.

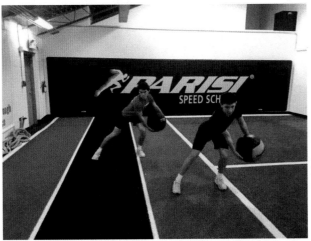

Will and Dan Parisi med ball training at Parisi Speed School.

First, this kind of training increases the development of motor engrams, the neurological "motor-skill programs" that coordinate the recruiting, synchronizing, and firing of your muscles and connective tissues to efficiently maximize power production. That's a skill you can develop and improve for any movement.

When you're training with an isokinetic form of resistance, the more force you put into it, the more resistance it's going to give back. And when you maximize your efforts all the way through the power stroke with that kind of modality, you're recruiting more motor engram units at every stage and generating more force in the process. With weight training, your force production is *decreasing* at the end ranges of your motion. Because you're no longer trying to accelerate the weight. You're decelerating it at the end of the movement to control the momentum required to lift it. And the end range of motion is the most important part of the lift. You want to be able to explode through it. That's why Louie Simmons and the guys at Westside Barbell in Columbus, Ohio, originally started the now-popular use of putting chains and bands on weightlifting bars to increase resistance at the end range of motion. This approach is scientifically proven[20] to enhance strength, power, and explosiveness because you are able to accelerate the bar through more of the full range of motion.

Second, with accommodating isokinetic resistance, you have the ability to create greater co-contractions. The co-contraction of muscles as they shorten and lengthen increases their girth. This stretches the fascia wrapping around it, which translates to greater force transmission. This concept is known as "hydraulic amplitude." One of the experts who really helped me understand this dynamic is Tom Findley, MD, Ph.D., co-founder of the Fascia Research Society. I'll try to explain the principle using a food analogy, since I'm Italian. Imagine squeezing a sausage. As you squeeze it, a section will get fatter. As this happens, the fascia-like wrapping surrounding that section will stretch and then return to its original shape.

This is what happens to your fascia when you co-contract muscles using natural resistance. The girth of the muscle group increases and stretches the fascia, which creates greater force transmission for that contraction as the muscle returns to its original length.

Frans Bosch is another world-renowned speed coach I had the privilege of talking to about the subject recently. Frans doesn't typically prescribe traditional heavy lifting for his athletes. Everything he does is built around co-contractions and executing each exercise with high speeds all the way to the very end range of motion. This is virtually impossible to do with traditional weight training (except for Olympic lifts). Frans prescribes a host of unique exercise movements that take advantage of natural forms of resistance to enforce these principles.

This runs contrary to the popular concept that heavy weight training will increase speed. The notion that heavy weight training can increase speed originally gained momentum in the wake of a groundbreaking Harvard University study[21] published in 2000 by human locomotion expert and biomechanist Peter Weyand, Ph.D.. In that study, Peter determined that the swing time of the recovery leg was virtually the same for both super-fast athletes and slower athletes alike, but that super-fast athletes have the ability to generate more force into the ground than slower athletes. In fact, he found that the force super-fast athletes apply into the ground on average during each foot strike is up to 2.5 times their body weight, while slower amateur athletes generate only an average force of 1.8 times their body weight during each foot strike.

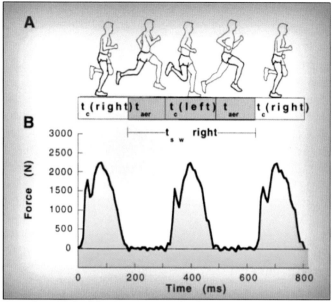

A study published by Peter Weyand, Ph.D., in 2000 revealed that force generation is the key to speed.

This means that a super-fast 150-pound athlete can generate an average force of 375-pounds down into the ground during each foot strike compared to a slower athlete of the same weight (who only generates approximately 275-pounds of force). This is referred to as "mass-specific force," and it means that the more force you can develop and put into the ground relative to your body weight, the faster you will run.

After Peter's study hit the press in 2000, much of the industry started to focus on lifting heavy weights under the assumption that getting stronger would make you faster. It makes sense on the surface. In theory, the stronger you are the more force you can generate into the ground and the faster you will run.

For weaker, early stage athletes with a young training age this holds true. Because most of these early strength gains are more neurological and coordination based. But as an athlete matures and develops more strength, the continued gains begin to fade quickly. Soon, many strength coaches were promoting the concept that you don't need to run to get fast. You just need to get strong. Which just sounded crazy to me. Because I know that all athletes need a balanced approach to training. It wasn't until 10 years later, in 2010, that Peter Weyand and his colleagues did a second study on this subject. The 2010 study[22] showed that it not only was the amount of mass-specific vertical force that subjects could apply to the ground, but also how rapidly this force could be applied (i.e. minimum ground contact time), that determined top speed in several types of gaits including forward and backward running, and one-leg hopping.

Then in 2014, Ken Clark, Ph.D., a former Parisi Speed School athlete who trained in our program as a high school student in Connecticut and studied under Peter during his doctoral program at SMU—which has the best human locomotion laboratory in the United States—conducted a groundbreaking study[23] in which he and Peter took a closer look at the foot-strike force signatures of world class sprinters and compared them to amateur field-sport athletes. In this study, the researchers noticed the force signatures of elite sprinters were noticeably different compared to those of amateur runners. While the force signatures of amateur athletes showed a more symmetrical bell curve, elite sprinters had an asymmetrical shape with a noticeable spike of force production at the very beginning of ground contact.

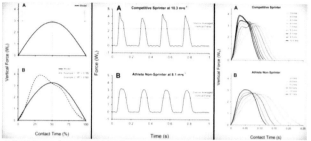

A 2014 study at SMU by Peter Weyand and Ken Clark revealed that elite runners have a very unique force signature as compared to amateur field sport athletes.

This was the case when elite sprinters ran at the same speeds as the amateurs, and it became more pronounced at faster speeds. One reason for this is that world class sprinters hit the ground with a much stiffer lower leg compared to amateur field sport athletes, because slower athletes leak energy by not having the ability to co-contract and stiffen their lower leg during ground contact.

In addition to being neurological, I believe this ability is also very much fascia based. Because fascia helps facilitate co-contraction. Not only does the lower leg have to be stiffer at ground contact for maximum force and speed, but the entire core and hip complex needs to be stiffer at ground contact. This stiffness is facilitated by co-contractions of the fascia system that minimizes energy leaks up the entire kinetic chain.

Of course, as soon as we got one of Dave's first isokinetic machines, I reached out to Ken Clark, who is now a professor at West Chester University's Exercise Science Lab, and arranged a study comparing the force signatures generated by Dave's machine against a traditional trap bar deadlift. In those studies, using the same bar speeds for the trap bar and the isokinetic machine, the data showed that a traditional trap bar deadlift creates a very choppy force signature.

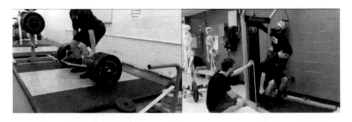

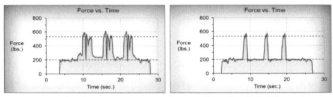

Comparing the force signatures of a trap bar deadlift (L) vs. the OHM machine (R) with Ken Clark at West Chester University's Exercise Science Lab.

This is because your force production decreases as the bar gains momentum. At the top of the motion, you begin to decelerate and slow the weight down. No matter how much weight you're lifting, there's momentum carrying that weight up or riding with it down. So, there's always an eccentric deceleration phase. In contrast, the force signature with the OHM machine was always very crisp, clean, and straight. It went straight up through the full range of motion. That type of force signature is much more aligned with how an athlete jumps, runs, and throws. And when you train that way using your whole body, you're increasing motor engram development and tissue recruitment in ways that directly translate to better force production at the very end range of your output, where it matters most. By my math, that makes Dave's mission to develop an athletic training modality that replicates natural physics an unprecedented success. But, as he is quick to point out, there are significant differences between the '80s-era isokinetic technology of the Leaper (which has since faded away in the marketplace) and the 21st century technology of Dave's equipment, which he refers to as "delta-kinetic."

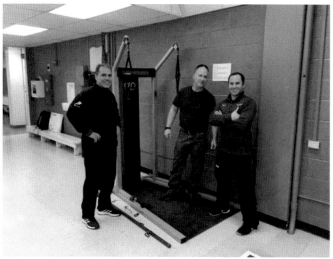

Conducting force plate studies of an early OHM machine with Dave Schmidt (C), and Ken Clark (R) at the West Chester University Exercise Science Lab.

"It's a brand-new term I've trademarked," Dave explains. "But it's an accurate way of defining how humans move. Everything we do is based on variable force and variable speed. I describe our equipment as being delta kinetic because it allows you to move freely against an isokinetic medium. Since it's motorized, it's already in motion when you engage it. So anybody can start pushing or pulling against it with minimal force and go as hard or soft as they want to. It provides variable resistance and variable speed based on your input, because that's human motion. Human motion is delta kinetic."

Here's the thing: Where I come from, we don't care what you call it. We just care if it works. As the headquarters for an international athletic franchise with world-class pedigree, the Parisi Speed School in Fair Lawn is approached on a near-weekly basis by new fitness equipment and product manufacturers who want us to use their latest thing. They often have clever marketing names and dazzling descriptions, but all we care about is: Does it work? Show us the data. Probably around 95 percent of them don't make the cut. But the first time I got on one of Dave's machines, I knew he was onto something. It was like the Leaper, but a 21st century version. I could rip through all kinds of different motions with it—throwing, lifting, pushing, running—and give 100 percent of my effort all the way to the end of the motion. It even provided me with visual feedback on digital displays that showed my real-time force output along with my left/right imbalances and more. My mind was blown. After convincing Dave to leave two of his beta units with us, I asked our coaching staff to incorporate them into their training for a month or so and report back. I mostly tell this story because the owner of our Fair Lawn facility—Rich Sadiv—is not only a world-class masters weight lifter with multiple titles who has deadlifted 640 pounds at a bodyweight of 198 pounds at the age 54. He also has one of the best bullshit meters of anyone I know. Rich is not only immune to the flashy whiz-bang of marketing hype, he is openly critical of anything that smells even remotely like it. But I'm going to stop gesturing intensely with my fork and let Dave tell this story, because I think it was more interesting from where he sat. Also, I finished my salad like four paragraphs ago.

"OK. Sure. I'll admit it. Having someone at the Parisi Speed School understand what I created was pretty inspiring. But Northern Jersey boys aren't easily persuaded in general. And Rich cuts a pretty intimidating figure. His first reaction was basically, 'You know what? I lift weights. That's my sport. I can't see myself ever really using this thing.' Then you, being the coach you are, said, 'Hey guys, huddle up here real fast! I want to ask all of you, whether you like it or not, to please use this thing for a few weeks and report back on the results. That's all I ask.' So I left two of our prototypes at the facility to see how it went. I honestly didn't know what to expect. When I returned to get their feedback, I was pleased to hear the first coach—the facility director and former New York Giants strength and conditioning coach, Craig Stoddard—get up and say, 'I gotta tell you guys—this thing is pretty incredible. I've been using it with a 12-year-old disabled girl who's recovering from cancer. She's got some significant physical imbalances. She can't even lift our weights. But when she gets on this equipment, she feels like a rock star. Her parents came to me the other day to say that her self-esteem is way up, and she looks forward to coming to the gym now.'

"Of course, that was a wonderful thing to hear as an inventor. But then the next coach stepped up and said 'Well my story's a little different. I've been training a number of the New York Jets and Giants guys. These guys are absolute animals, but it's just kicking their butts. They're pushing upwards of 400 pounds on it and loving the experience and seeing some great results!'

"Then Rich finally steps up and reluctantly admits, 'All right, so I did use this thing and I'm surprised to say it actually works.

69

I've cut down my traditional lifting and I'm now up 3 percent in how much I can lift in just over three weeks.'

"To see a guy like Rich take to it was a big win for me. Now he's hitting some of his all-time best marks in the bench press at 54 years old—a point in life where he told me he only expected to see his numbers going down—and I believe it's because our equipment allows him to train by pushing with optimal force all the way through his full range of motion. Now he can safely work his entire chest and core all the way down through his feet with a much lower risk of injury compared to traditional weight training. This allows him to build up his stabilizing connective tissues and muscles while also proprioceptively training his nervous system for a more balanced movement sequence. So, when he finally does lie down to push up on an actual weight, he's able to push it with greater efficiency and more stable force production."

It's at this point—looking out from the edge of the continent at the fiery hues of a setting sun—that I remember I'm talking to the inventor of a new technology most people have never heard of about how to train a virtually invisible biological system with huge potential that has been largely overlooked for as long as we've been training athletes. I can hear the waves below mixing with the distant sound of a bouncing medicine ball and the buzzing fluorescent lights of a high school gym. I begin seeing the different puzzle pieces of my past and future coming together from around the globe to create a new, more highly evolved approach to improving human performance.

And it occurs to me that someone should write a book about it.

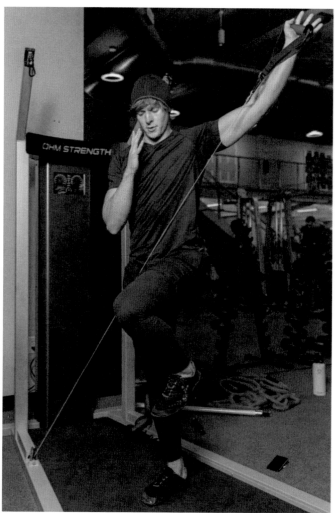

Credit: Jonathan Cunningham.

Mechanical Composites: The Science of Speed and Power

REMEMBER WHEN I MADE THAT JOKE about Tom Myers having "forgotten more about the fascia system than I will ever know?" Yeah, I was only half kidding about that. While I often can't find my car keys (especially if I'm running more than 10 minutes late), I get the feeling Tom still remembers what he ate for lunch in 5th grade. That dude's mind is a steel trap. But you know who actually *has* forgotten more about the fascia system than I will probably ever know? Dr. Stuart McGill, a quick-witted, bushy-mustached former kinesiology professor from Canada who has authored multiple books and published more research papers than he can count (the actual number is somewhere north of 240) over the course of the his 30-plus years running the Spinal Biomechanics Lab and Back Pain Clinic at the University of Waterloo. During his tenure, he studied animals, cadavers, students, professional athletes, and whatever else he could get his hands on, asking deep questions, analyzing raw data, crunching the numbers, doing the hard science, and coming to non-negotiable, research-based conclusions about how the body works to produce power and reduce injury.

This is why he's flown around the world to serve as an expert speaker, consultant, trainer, and back injury recovery specialist (aka: Dr. Back Mechanic) to some of the world's most elite athletes. Like, seriously, the kind of athletes he could only name if he killed you afterwards.

This is also why I've collaborated with Stu to refine the Parisi Speed School methodology and have invited him to speak at various conferences I've hosted for the NFL's Professional Football Strength and Conditioning Coaches Association (PFSCA). That's how we ended up in a spirited conversation one night on a hotel balcony at Red Rock Resort, overlooking the outskirts of Las Vegas, when some of the biggest pieces of the fascia training puzzle snapped together for me.

It all started with a question. After dedicating more than three decades of his life to creating his own biomechanics lab, educating thousands of students, mentoring dozens of grad students-turned-professors, and working with some of the most powerful superhumans society has ever produced, Stu retired from his professorship at the university to spend more time with his family and explore bigger, bolder, more practical ideas.

On the day he retired, he literally walked away from his lab, inviting his grad students and fellow researchers to come take whatever equipment and research materials they wanted. In the relatively conservative "ride-'til-you-die" world of academia, it was kind of a punk rock thing to do. Looking out on the distant shining skyline of Sin City, I had to ask: What drove him to do that?

"Many of my questions came from working with the superstars," Stu says. "I wanted to know what made them a superstar. Why can they do that? What can I measure? But academic research is built around creating statistical models and studying one animal.

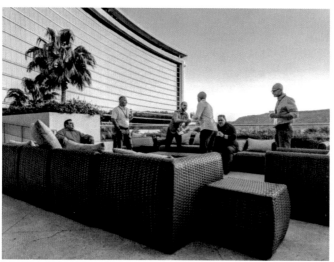

Meet and Greet for NFL strength and conditioning coaches at the 2018 PFSCA Injury Resiliency Conference on a sunset patio deck at Red Rock Resort in Nevada. Credit: Johnathon Allen.

"That means you have to measure 20 people to reach statistical significance. Well that only works if you have 20 identical animals. And the human condition is highly variable. There are total beasts and there are complete sloths. It's a highly variable, non-homogeneous system. Reaching statistical significance is irrelevant to me. I don't care about the average. I care about variability—my whole world is about variability. Not only are there differences in performance variables but also in injury resilience, responses to treatment, and training. I remember one athlete who got sliced up by an outboard propeller in an accident. "Yet he could still run and create fantastic amounts of force. How was that possible? Well, it was because of his fascia. But it was those kinds of questions that would prompt my colleagues to look at me and ask, 'Why do you hang around with coaches and athletes?'

"Well, it's because I want to work with the human Ferraris. And I get to ask such interesting questions. It's just how I roll. And man—some of the Ferraris I've driven—if only I could tell you the stories. Some of them are just ungodly creatures. But many of my peers were still teaching students that muscles are agonists or antagonists. And I fought with myself for years over teaching these very junior concepts that really do nothing to enhance performance and reduce injuries. In fact, I would argue they inhibit understanding."

When I asked Stu to explain that idea and how it related to my current topic of interest—the fascia system—his eyes lit up with a hundred thoughts all happening at once, each racing to get in front of the other.

"How about this?" Stu said in his professor voice. "As you know, I like to structure discussions around a scientific principle and then talk about how those principles apply in the practical world—so, in this case, how they would apply to a coach's world. Sound good?"

I subconsciously nod, because of course I do. I also pull out my iPhone, hit record, and set it on the table.

"OK, well, talking in terms of the fascia system, connective tissues, injury resilience, and performance, let's just start by thinking about this idea of muscles being agonists and antagonists. If you're performing a biceps curl, most people would argue that the biceps is an agonist and the triceps is an antagonist, right? Well I just felt awful teaching first-year students that concept in my later years. I would say to them, 'This is so simplistic! Sure, it'll help you pass your mid-term in two months, but it's nowhere close to what goes on in the body.' I mean, consider the hamstring muscle in sprinting. You might say the hamstring forms an eccentric breaking action at the hip and knee at a certain phase of the sprint cycle just before heal strike. Now consider getting out of a chair or performing a squat. That same hamstring muscle extends the hip—which you have to do in order to get up from a squat—but it also flexes the knee, which collapses the squat. That muscle is now helping at one joint and collapsing in the other joint. So, if I asked you: What's the agonist here? Do you see how silly it is to even begin that discussion? The concept of agonists and antagonists would work only if there were no fascia, and you just had a single joint muscle. But most of the muscles in the body are multi-articular. They cross several joints. And they're all surrounded and integrated with fascia, which is a mechanical connection that creates a crosstalk of forces throughout the body.

"Now consider the spine. If you do a dead lift, or run, or jump, or throw a javelin, all the muscles in the torso are active. What's the agonist and what's the antagonist? The front of the torso is active, the back is active, the sides are active. Every single muscle in the torso is an agonist to throwing the javelin. And I would argue that if they weren't, you'd be open to injury. So, that's my opening principle—that this model of agonists and antagonists falls apart when we understand the system as a mechanical composite."

And there it was again—that metaphor—flashing across the desert sky: "mechanical composite," "tensegrity model," "symphony of systems" ... all expressions of the same idea coming together from some of the brightest minds I know, to create a new constellation of biomechanical understanding.

So, I asked him to explain what he means by "mechanical composite."

"If I gave you a piece of maple wood, you could measure its strength and stiffness. Now imagine I took that same piece of maple and cut it into veneers and cross-plied those veneers back together again with an adhesive layer. I don't contribute any more wood, but now it's *plywood*. And plywood is a mechanical composite. It's super stiff and super strong. That's what the body does. It's a mechanical composite. And that comes from the fascia, which allows our bodies to create springs that generate more force through the entire linkage of the whip action that you're creating when you throw a javelin. Those are foundational principles you can prove; they're measurable. I've done the experiments in rats with one of my students (Stephen Brown, now a professor of health and nutrition at the University of Guelph)[24]. We did surgeries where we kept the muscle tissues alive but separated them and removed the fascia and measured the change in force and stiffness, while keeping the other half of the torso muscles intact and measuring the super stiffness and the super strength. What we found was that when you take out the fascia, the total force that you measure from each muscle doesn't equal the sum of force that you measure on the intact side. That's because of the super stiffness and super strength that the fascia provides."

Hold up! Time out! I'm up to speed on Stu's research and principles around increasing power production by developing super strength and super stiffness in the core. They're well documented in his books[25] and presentations. We've made them a fundamental element of the Parisi Speed School. Core stiffness and stability are the foundation for all athletic performance.

Or, to put it another way: You can't shoot a canon from a canoe. Maintaining ultra-strong stiffness in the core of the body is what gives your arms and legs the rock-solid anchor they need to act as whips that transfer force through the linkage system of your body without leaking energy through the core. But this was the first time I could recall hearing Stu talk in such detail about how the fascia system factors into this dynamic, and I had no idea he'd done in-depth research specifically around that. To me this was a new, largely unexplored area of athletic science. So, I asked him why I hadn't come across his rat studies or other fascia-related research before.

"Well, Bill, you know I'm not allowed to do operations on humans and split their fascia," Stu says, smiling wryly. "And, honestly, I never thought in a million years anyone would ask me about this stuff again. I thought that when I retired from the university, no one would care, and I'd just go fishing or something. But, yes, back then I had to come up with animal models to answer some of these questions. So I teamed up with rat physiologists who would be probing how a certain diet might influence vascular health, for example, and then I'd get the rat at the end, and my team would perform the fascia-muscle work. But, really, I've been studying the role of the fascia system since back in the '80s. Back then, I would conduct a cadaver dissection and then do an MRI of a live person—because a cadaver has obviously shrunken and atrophied. I would get my geometry from the cadaver, and then I'd look at live humans—at athletes and non-athletes. I'd measure their muscle cross-sectional areas and fiber direction vectors. Then I'd put them on a dynamometer and measure their performance.

"What I found was that their strength and power were way higher than what was predicted by the size of their muscles measured from MRI. I couldn't understand it. I said to myself, 'What the hell am I missing?' Again, this is back in the '80s, when you were probably still throwing javelins at Iona. That's when I started to understand what was happening.

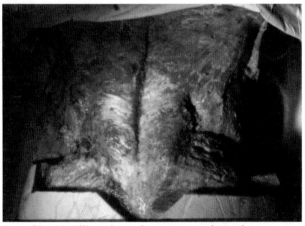

One of Stu McGill's cadaver dissections studying the interconnections of fascia and muscle tissue in the core. Credit Stu McGill.

"For example, when you do a sit-up, anatomy textbooks will say that *rectus abdominis* flexes the torso, right? Well, when I measured athletes doing a sit-up, less than 20 percent of the flexor power came from their *rectus*. Not even a fifth!

"Where was the other 81 percent coming from? It was coming from the abdominal wall— transmitted through the fascia. *Rectus abdominis* has a beaded architecture. It has a contractile component, and then a lateral tendon, and then a contractile component, another cross tendon, and so on. That series of beads forms the six pack.

"Those tendons crossing laterally through *rectus abdominis* have heavy fascia connections above and below, both superficial and deep. And that's all connected to the abdominal wall. "It's the oblique muscles that create all those fascial forces and then fuse into the *rectus*. The *rectus* is really an anchor for the abdominal wall, and the abdominal wall is so much bigger than the *rectus*. Go measure a really strong dude. You'll find they've got big oblique muscles— they're three centimeters thick on some of those people. Remember, it's about strength from the core. We keep coming back to that."

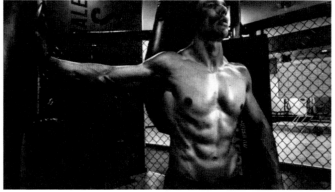

Super strength and super stiffness are enabled by the anchor of a strong core. Source: PXHere.

That's when I realized I had actually grabbed my mug (technically, it was a glass of unsweetened iced tea) and leaned in.

"And this segues nicely back to my second point," Stu continues, "which is that when a muscle contracts, it creates force. But it also creates stiffness. When you throw a javelin, you need muscle force to initiate the movement.

But, as you know, when a muscle is fully hard and contracted, it won't move, because it's so stiff. Then the pulse comes, and hopefully you've stored some elastic energy, so you can release that spring. But if you keep the muscle force high, you'll never release any energy. So there's this interplay between force and stiffness.

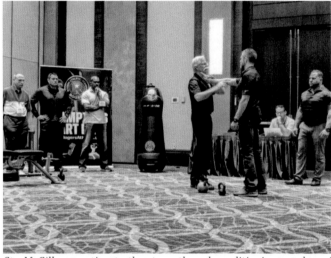

Stu McGill presenting to the strength and conditioning coaches of the NFL. Credit: Johnathon Allen.

"If you were to stand up right now, I could teach you to stand with virtually no effort using a very balanced muscle system. But are you standing because your muscles are creating force? Or because they're contracting and stiffening the joints, which allows you to stack your mass and stand tall? What you'll find is that it's less about muscle force and more about muscle *stiffness*.

"To put this into terms you can relate to as a coach, think of a collision on the football field.

The question in this situation might be, should we strengthen the players' necks? A strength and conditioning coach might argue that you can reduce a player's risk of concussion and cervical spine injury by doing neck-strengthening exercises. Well, neck strength has less to do with it. What you're creating is a *system of stiffness*. If you get cracked in the head, helmet-to-helmet, the muscles turn on to create stiffness—stop the rotation, stop the concussion, and stop the strain. Because it's strain that damages tissue. It's not load, it's not rate of force development, it's strain to the tissue—deformation."

So, how does that apply to fascia training? I was just thinking the same thing. Luckily, it was a warm spring night, and the neon-tinged sky was filling with stars. I could tell Stu had his story-telling mustache on, and we were just getting to the third act. I set my now-empty glass down on the table, checked to make sure the phone was still recording, and fired off that very question.

"Well, this is all part and parcel with muscle activation and how it interacts with fascia. I've already argued that it's very difficult to go with this agonist/antagonist model. But what fascia does by putting compression nets around all of your muscles, is that it turns *every* muscle into an agonist.

"If I were to cut one of the heads of your hamstrings, we'd have three heads of hamstrings. If we cut one of them halfway through, what you'd notice is that—once it heals from the trauma—you won't lose half the strength of that muscle. Even though you've cut it halfway through, you'll only lose a little bit. That's because all of the muscle fibers that were cut in half are still connected through the fascia. They may no longer go tendon to tendon, but they go from the tendon through the fascia covering the muscle, and they bypass the cut. But if you were sitting on a knee flexion machine, and we could very precisely control and measure your knee flexor force, what you'd notice is that if you cut away the fascia from around the hamstrings, you would lose a *lot* of strength. Because the forces in the hamstrings are really just tightening and tuning the fascia around the quads—that's what super-strengthens, and super-stiffens them."

I was feeling pretty good about keeping up with a guy like Stu on this whole concept of the fascia system being a mechanical composite that creates a neurologically responsive system of stiffness that enables mobility, amplifies force, and protects us from injury. So I chimed in with some of my thoughts on the kangaroo study because, you know—kangaroos.

Then I realized Stu was already four hops ahead of me.

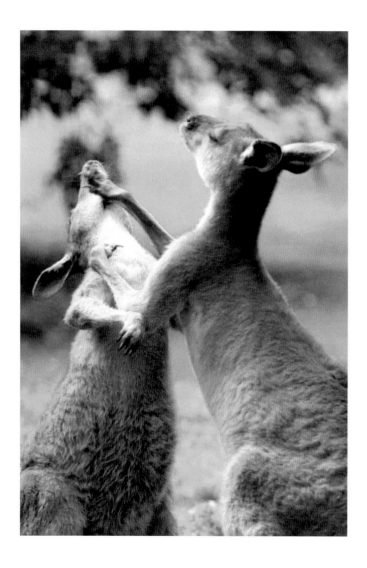

"Oh, yes! I used to use some of those textbooks by McNeil Alexander[26]. He's a fabulous zoological bio-mechanist. He studied wallabies, kangaroos, elephants, giraffes—looking at their systems and how they all worked. I believe it was he and his graduate students who documented the energy expenditure of kangaroos. He had kangaroos walking and hopping along with gas masks on, so he could figure out their oxygen use and that sort of thing. An amusing side note to that study is that it turns out kangaroos use much more energy just slowly plodding along, walking on their big goofy feet, than they do when they're storing and converting elastic energy bounding along in hops. When they're bounding, they inject a tiny little muscle pulse that loads the spring through a controlled muscle contraction and then lets the spring release that energy. The muscle isn't there to create force and length change. The muscle, integrated with the fascia, is turned into a spring that is precisely tuned from neural activation to effectively store then release the spring energy. And that is exactly how great players dunk a basketball!"

It's worth pausing this conversation to clarify that there are many different body types—or as I like to think of them, human animal types—some more fascia-based in their movement strategies and others more muscle-based. Some have spines that function like flexible whips, others are stiff like logs. There are also different sports, positions, goals, and activities that require very specific body types, movement proficiencies, and motor engram literacies. With all of that said, I asked Stu if he had any suggestions or general recommendations for training the fascia system.

"One recommendation I would make is to be careful with things like stretching. We don't stretch to create mobility, but that idea is so ingrained in American training culture. You won't find it as influential in the Russian and European performance cultures. You can use stretching to tune your fascia system and get it to play with the neurology of the pulse-and-release of elastic energy. But if you stretch fascia elastics away, all you're left with is muscle. And then you've lost your spring, you've lost endurance, and you wear out faster in endurance events. The body responds to specific stimulation. When you put a lot of load through the body, the tissues adapt to become stiffer. When you lay down more bone, it gets stiffer. When you build more muscle strength and support for the joints, they become stiffer. In contrast, if all you do is yoga and you avoid load, you lose that stiffness, which in scientific language we call compliance. But spring energy is half K-X squared, with K being spring stiffness and X being the distance that spring has stretched, squared. When a function is squared, small differences matter. If you are a yogi, not only do you lose the ability to produce, store, and recover athletic force, but your body also changes. It loses tissue resiliency. So, it will allow extreme postures, and strain more easily. And, as I mentioned before, it's *strain*—deformation at the molecular level of the tissues—that causes tears, fractures, evulsions, and all the rest. Of course, I'm talking in the extremes of, say, an Olympic weightlifter versus someone doing yoga. Golf is really closer to the mobility spectrum where you want to develop a finely tuned fascia system. In that sport, you want the body to be a spring, not a log. If you use too much muscle when you're trying to golf, you'll find the ball doesn't go very far.

"That's because the stiffness created by muscle contraction overpowers the force and slows you down. You ruin the release of energy that creates the elastic whip.

"Another thing I would say is that it's important not to confuse the tissue adaptation process. For example, if you're lifting with maximal effort one day, and then you go out and try to play golf or throw a javelin the next, you're confusing those tissue adaptations. One day, you're telling them to stiffen up as much as possible—to hold the tissues as tightly as they can to provide maximum resilience—and then the next day, you're telling them to go out and be a spring. Well, you've just confused the whole adaptation process of those tissues. Everything is a compromise. And when I hear people say they're going for 100 percent strength; my response is that your tissues need to *earn* that. You've got to earn the capacity to train at a 100 percent. In fact, I would advise nearly every athlete against it, unless it is pulsed strength.

"Let me wrap this up with a story. One of my clients was one of the world's best marathoners. Of course, he came to me with back pain. As you know, that's really why anyone comes to me. But when they come, I can't be neglectful of what else I can do to enhance their performance. That's the trick of it all—when I can do both. So I always say to them, OK, we're going to do these things for your back, but if I were a genie, and could grant you one athletic wish, what would it be? I don't want to be boastful, but the truth is that I can usually achieve it. In this case, this marathoner said, 'The worst part of my race is the first two miles. I'm slow. So, I end up having to create a mental and physical strategy to catch up, so I can win back what I lost in the first two miles.'

"Right away I said, well, show me your warmup. So he went to the wall and did a runner's stretch—stretching his Achilles tendon. And I said, OK, what *else* do you do? Then he did another isometric stretch and a little light jog and lined up to the starting line. He was doing *nothing* to potentiate his body. He was just doing things to de-tune himself, put his neurology to sleep, and ruin his springs. So I said, humor me. For your next warmup, start by doing mobility drills that involve no stretching at all. Just work through your range of motion, but don't go near the end of the range. Go to 95 percent, but don't stay there. Don't stretch. Just mobilize your tissues, round out your joints, take out the stress risers. Then move to potentiate and prime your physiology. Get your heart rate up. Get your hormone levels where they need to be for the run. Then, third, focus on your neural priming. Tune your muscles. Tune the springs. Tune the neurology. I'm not kidding, Bill, he not only went out and won his next race, he ran the fastest first two miles he'd ever run. And all we did was potentiate his body rather than put his fascia and neurology to sleep. How's that for a story?"

BOOM! Did you hear that? It was like a mic drop with a dozen shooting stars exploding over Las Vegas all at once (relax, people—it was just an iced tea)! It's just that I've known Stu for a number of years. I've heard him give amazing talks on a wide range of topics, but I've never heard him tell these stories or explain in such detail how the fascia system fits into athletic performance. Turns out all I had to do was ask. And suddenly, the puzzle pieces from decades of research and experience all came snapping together.

Bill Parisi / Johnathon Allen

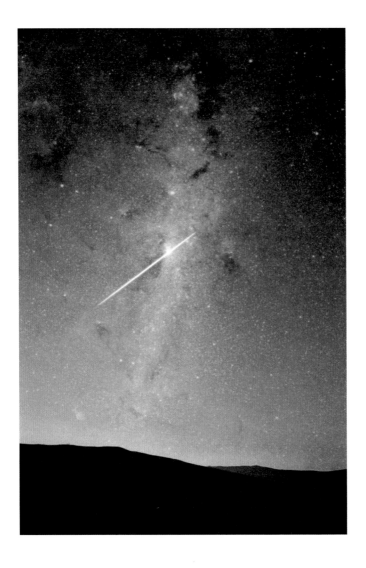

The Art of Coaching: Mailboxes, and Mechanotransduction

AS PREVIOUSLY MENTIONED, one of the best things about this lifelong quest I'm on is that now I get to explore it at the highest levels. Years of hard work, experience, training, and curiosity have paid off. Succeeding in my goal to help athletes of all ages and types achieve their maximum potential—to not just win, but to realize their full athletic capabilities—has given me the opportunity to interact with a global community of other like-minded professionals who have mentored and coached some of the most remarkable athletes of our time. This means that after I have a paradigm-shifting conversation with a super-smart guy like Stu McGill that keeps me up half the night buzzing with a mind full of unanswered questions, I can wake up the next day and continue that conversation with other super-smart guys, like internationally renowned coach, Dan Pfaff. To put this in scale for you folks keeping score at home, Dan has coached 49 Olympians (including 10 medalists), more than 50 World Championship competitors (nine medalists), and five world-record holders. And we're just getting started. He's also helped athletes achieve more than 55 national records, served on the coaching staffs of five Olympic Games in five different countries and ... yeah, you get the idea. The dude knows some things. And when you've helped hang that much hardware around that many necks, people listen to what you have to say.

This is why I invited him to the PFSCA conference in Las Vegas to present to the strength and conditioning coaches of the NFL alongside Stu and a panel of other experts on the subject of improving injury resilience and recovery. When I saw Dan enjoying the scenic morning view from the same deck where Stu and I had had our conversation the night before, I grabbed my mug of coffee and wandered over to get his take on the subject of fascia training and how it applies in the real world.

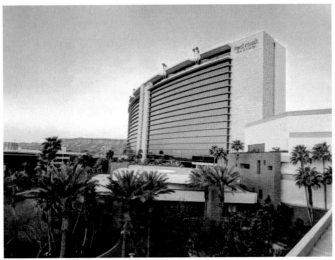

Sunrise at Red Rock Resort in Nevada.
Credit: Johnathon Allen.

"Well, at the end of the day, training is a matter of introducing mechanical factors into the body," Dan replies from under a somewhat less bushy, less grey mustache. "But what's happening in the body involves a spectrum of factors. So, if you use a heavy load and go slowly, that's creating certain responses. If you use a light load and go really fast, that's creating other responses. It's the same thing with energy systems.

You can't really train energy systems in an isolated sequential manner, because the moment you start moving, all the energy systems are at play. It's a matter of which one's predominating in the activity. That applies to muscle systems, fascia systems, and so on. Any movement, just being alive, is creating a training effect. It's how we manipulate and shift the stressor of that information—that's when you get into the specifics of training. But I think it would be a misnomer to say that we're just training fascia, because that's impossible."

Man, what a bull's-eye. The thing is, we live in a culture where people like to think in terms of absolutes. We want to simplify things and reduce them to the "one way" or the "best way." But the reality is that you're never just training the aerobic system, or the ATP-PC system, or the muscle system, or the fascia system. They're all being trained all the time. It's a question of what level each system is being trained at.

That said, our understanding of how the body's fascia system adapts, tunes, and remodels itself is still a young science with tremendous potential. So, I asked Dan to explain a little bit about his understanding of fascia tissue, fibroblast activity, and how they factor into training programs for different kinds of athletes.

"Fibroblasts are part of a communication system within the collagen matrix that's independent but runs in parallel with the central nervous system. A lot of the proprioceptive research that's been done is just looking at a central nervous system-only communication system. Where, in fact, it's deeply embedded and entwined into this collagen matrix communication system in which fibroblasts serve as a major antenna, receiver, and speaker.

"The fundamental principal in all of this is a term called mechanotransduction. So, whether you're doing movement exercises or rehab therapies or what have you, it all circles back to introducing mechanotransduction factors into the system to create change."

Quick primer on fibroblasts and mechanotransduction: As I mentioned earlier, fibroblast cells are the architects of the fascia system. Basically, when fascia tissue is exposed to impact, vibration, pressure, or stress, an electrical charge is generated in the fascia tissue matrix that causes fibroblast cells to go to that spot and start producing collagen and other molecules as needed along those lines of stress, vibration, and impact.

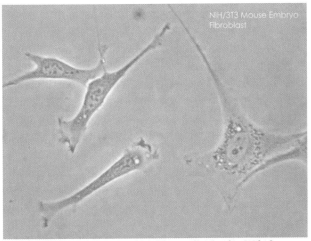

NIH/3T3 mouse tissue fibroblast cells. Credit: Wikidata.

"Mechanical action transduces information into the system—whether it's rubbing, or pressing, or moving—and the system has to react to that information," Dan replies.

"If I've got a knot in my leg and I rub on it, that's a mechanical action. And all of the structures—the fascia, the muscle, lymph system, vessel system, and everything else—are going to react accordingly to that mechanical stress. So the speed of the mechanical input, the force of the mechanical input, the vectors and angles of that input are all going to result in a unique reaction.

"In terms of elastic training, where you're challenging the collagen matrix—whether it be tendons, ligaments, bursa, fat pads, or fascia—with exercise menu items that are skewed towards that part of the spectrum, there are going to be multiple layers of complexity in that outcome. Slow, non-forceful inputs at a certain angle are going to result in a movement solution for that input. Likewise, bigger, faster, more forceful movements are going to result in a different movement solution appropriate for those inputs. It's all influenced by the dynamics of the input."

The question I keep coming back to is, how do we use this knowledge to better inform our training approach for different athletes? Dan has worked with virtually every type of athlete there is. Obviously, they each require different approaches. Some are more fascia-based, some are more muscle-based. Two examples are Ameer Webb and Andre DeGrasse—both sprinters that Dan has worked with who have very different body types. So, I asked him how he approaches training for those two different kinds of animals.

"Well, it's hard to get into simplifications. I would say that their movement solution preference is one of the many factors that we look at when we're designing their programs. If you have an athlete who tends to rely more on their fascia structures and capabilities versus a person who favors muscular solutions, then, yes, there are differences in the types of work and the magnitude of work that you would consider. But there are also all of these other variables at play, like volume and intensity, work-to-rest ratios, density patterns, how frequently you entertain a training menu item, and so on. That's why it's really important that we fight this tendency towards reductionism. Some athletes might be more fascia-inclined in certain types of movements or in states of fatigue, but in other states of movement or in a state of freshness, they may rely on different parts of their spectral drivers for activity. You have to remember these things operate spectrally. So, the question you're asking is, do you train a fascia-biased athlete differently than a slow-twitch-dominant athlete? Well I think, in a big rock sense, if you have an athlete who tends to rely more on fascia-driven movement solutions, and you train them to have a more muscular solution, then you're driving them away from their genetic homeostasis. You're diminishing their ability to use fascia solutions and biasing their options."

I find this idea of biasing movement options intriguing, so I ask him to explain it more.

"Well, movement bias is an important factor in all of this, because we have short memory systems. For example, if you're doing a big block of strength training, that becomes very familiar to you. So, you're going to default to that movement solution if you're under pressure or unsure. Now you've biased the cognitive perceptive desires towards strength rather than elasticity. If you've ever flown to England and rented a car where you have to drive on the other side of the road, you'll understand what bias is about.

"Part of our problem in writing programming or deciding what, when, and how to do it is that we need to categorize things or create some sort of flow chart to manage the massive amount of information and number of variables involved," Dan continues. "I think coaches, especially coaches who've been in the trenches for a while, tend to mailbox athletes. So, you might mailbox them by what sport they play, their position, their age, or their injury factors. Whether it's right or wrong, we mailbox people to simplify the training process and make more efficient programs. Hopefully, in this day and age, you wouldn't have your defensive and offensive linemen doing 5K runs through the woods in the off-season, because we know their bodies, joints, and mental wellness would rebel against that. My suggestion is, why not add another layer to the flow chart of how you mailbox people? So, sure, you could say everybody's going to work on a certain menu item, but how you work on it is going to differentiate for each individual based on their movement preferences and drivers. You're going to get more buy-in that way. Which means you're going to get a better harmonic and better reaction to the work."

This is a key point I think a lot of coaches and trainers forget when they're developing programming. Athletes, especially high-performance athletes, have a much better intuitive understanding of their bodies and what works for them than most coaches give them credit for. They know if the training they're doing makes sense to their bodies or doesn't. And—as noted in the title of this book—there are a tremendous number of interconnected systems involved in the production of human power and motion that function spectrally (cue the harmonic symphony).

There is no one size that fits all. But there are ways to develop and refine specific training menu items based on the animal and mailbox types you're dealing with. And that all starts with having a diverse collection of tools, experiences, and perspectives in your training tool kit.

"Again, I think the art of coaching is determining what problems an athlete is going to encounter in their sport or discipline. What are the big rocks? What are the essentials? What are the fundamentals? And then you work backwards from there to determine their individual KPIs—their key performance indicators. There are a lot of factors to consider. Depending on the athlete, they may be event-specific; they may be physiological; they may be training design; they could be mental factors; they could be environmental-life factors. There are a lot of factors. But we're primarily talking about programming and training. I've always operated on the principle that you should keep the strengths strong and slowly fill in the gaps on the weaknesses or deficiencies. That said, if you introduce a training menu item and stay with it for a while and see a negative trend occurring systemically across a lot of areas—and that's the number one variable you've adjusted—then you'd take it out and see if things clean up. A lot of it is just experimentation through time. But after you've done something enough times, you may start seeing patterns. You may see that certain body types struggle when you introduce certain menu items. So if you still think you need to introduce that thing, you may need to do it more slowly and less frequently and allow for a lot longer incubation period. Because if you try to mass jam something into the system, you'll get negative reactions all over the place.

"I think a lot of it is a matter of being really aware of how an athlete reacts to a change in their training formula or program. But it all starts with identifying the essentials and fundamentals for that individual, doing a KPI analysis and then creating a hierarchy for those KPIs before you begin to do the programming. You just have to remember that it's complex, spectral, and layered."

This is how you know you're dealing with an incredibly smart person: They can't be easily pinned down by generalizations. They recognize that—while our impulse is to simplify complex relationships in order to organize massive amounts of information—real life is highly variable, multilayered, and complex. With very smart people, the answer to almost every question is: "*It depends.*"

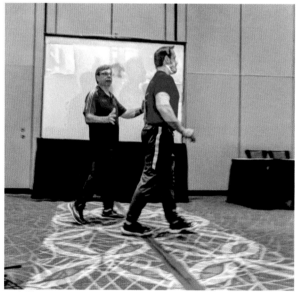

Dan Pfaff presenting to the strength and conditioning coaches of the NFL at the PFSCA Injury Resilience Conference.

"If you look at coaching or movement education, there are really two big rocks. There's physical literacy: Does the person have the basic components to execute the fundamental movement schemes? And then there's sport literacy: Can they take that physical literacy and convert it into usable time-force movement for the sport or task at hand? Our job as coaches is to ensure first and foremost that they have physical literacy, that they can do the fundamental movement patterns. Then, once they have a degree of mastery, we put additional stress on them by changing their environments or the nature of the tasks. Ultimately, that bleeds into the sport-specific layers. Take a sport like football. If you look at the sport literacy of a nose guard versus the sport literacy of a free safety—they're totally different packages. The next layer of classification is looking at what kind of person are you dealing with: What's their age, their training history, their injury history, their genetics, their body type, their perceptual skills, their drivers for being involved in sport? This is why I battle against reductionism and linear equation solutions in sport."

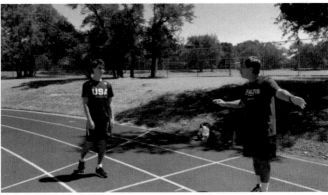

Will Parisi training with master coach Dan Pfaff in Austin, Texas.

Dovetailing with that, I ask Dan his opinion on doing things like training with ladder drills, which has become a hot topic of debate recently among coaches who think they're useless. For the record, I disagree. To me, they're just another tool in the training toolbox you can use to create specific inputs.

"Well ... *it depends*," Dan says with a cocked eye-brow and smile, as if he knew I knew he was going to say that.

"A menu apparatus like a ladder drill develops the physical literacy of certain joints, and postures, and rhythms. So, it may have value to an athlete who lacks physical literacy in some of those movement solutions. In which case, it has a positive effect. It'll give them context for a unique ground-contact time and air-time between contacts. But like any menu item, these things have a shelf life. If that's all you do— and you do a lot of it—then you're going to bias the system towards that activity. The detractors would say that when you sprint, there's big displacement. There's ascending flight time and descending contact time. Well, that's true. So, does a ladder drill teach you to sprint? No, but that's not why you would do it. Unfortunately, some coaches sell it that way. And I think that's why the critics exist. The way I try to explain it to young coaches is that, if you're a general contractor, when you get to the worksite in the morning, you'd better have a big toolbox with a lot of different tools. Because you've got a lot of puzzles to solve when you get out of that truck. You're going to have to deal with framing, electrical systems, plumbing, and cement work, and so on.

"The problem we have with a lot of coaching today is that people try to use the same tool for every job. Well, if I'm trying to pour a driveway and I've only got a hammer and a screwdriver, how am I going to smooth the concrete?"

I could keep having this conversation all day. But my mug is empty. The conference is about to start. And I just remembered I'm the one running it. So I have to rush off. Parting from Dan, I look up to see the pale silhouette of last night's moon still hanging over the desert mountains as a reminder.

The quest continues.

Deep Data: The Science of Coaching

AS THE FAMOUS STATISTICIAN, W. Edwards Deming, once said, "In God we trust, all others must bring data." Considering that Deming, an American engineer and management consultant, is regarded as having had a greater impact on Japanese society than any other person not from Japan (by helping the country rebuild from the nuclear ashes of WWII to become the second largest economy in the world in less than a decade), it's safe to say he understood the power of data. And many of his ideas—which coincidentally also support the importance of using a whole-system approach to improving performance— apply to athletic training as well as they do to manufacturing and business. To help athletes succeed, coaches and trainers need to be able to quickly make smart, data-driven decisions about what kind of person they're dealing with and what sort of training they need. That starts with having diagnostic tools that help you establish accurate baselines, metrics, and KPIs, for each animal, movement bias, and mailbox. That's why I'm flying cross country to Silicon Valley—the heart of American innovation—to meet with Dr. Phil Wagner, founder and CEO of Sparta Performance Science and developer of the Sparta Platform, a force plate that measures power output in the three distinct phases of a vertical jump—load, explode, and drive. Since its release in 2013, the Sparta Platform and its associated software have become a powerful diagnostic tool used by professional teams in every major sports franchise from the NFL to the NBA, MLB, NHL, and the rest of the alphabet—even the DOD.

107

Along the way, the Sparta Science™ database has accumulated more than one million anonymous scans (and growing), measuring the three-dimensional force signatures of athletes and non-athletes of every stripe. All of this jumping and scanning has led to the creation of what Dr. Wagner refers to as a well of "deep data" that provides remarkably accurate baselines for predicting injuries and measuring the success or failure of different training programs.

Fun fact about Dr. Wagner: In addition to being the CEO of a Silicon Valley tech startup and a professional strength and conditioning coach with multiple wins, the dude is also a certified medical doctor—as in "M.D." I'm going to do my level best not to call him "Dr. Phil" and ask him for relationship advice. It won't be easy.

"I originally went into the strength and conditioning profession with the idea of trying to help athletes avoid injuries, or at least reduce them, by using highly individualized data," says Phil. "But at the time, there weren't a lot of technologies available to do that.

"I thought, where is data and technology being used in the health sector right now? And it turned out that medical school was the best way for me to get that kind of education. So I approached USC, met with the dean, and explained, OK, I'm not going to practice medicine, but I can offer you some unique attributes by doing papers on biomechanics and collaborating with the physical therapy department. I ended up going through medical school for four years at USC while I was also working as a strength coach at UCLA. That gave me the unique opportunity to train as a physician while also working towards my end-goal of building a database that could be used to predict and reduce injuries for athletes. Essentially, I studied the processes involved in building databases for disease prediction and treatment. Probably one of the most common is diabetes, where you're figuring out, OK, what's a meaningful blood sugar level? And what are the best options for addressing that based on a person's age, ethnicity, and other factors? My idea was to take that model and apply it to athletics."

Sparta Science—which is located next door to Facebook in Menlo Park—is unlike any facility I've seen: part fitness gym, part human performance lab, part technology startup. Beyond the rows of weights, sleds, elastic bands, medicine balls, and foam rollers is a room full of software engineers and development strategists working away at computers and whiteboards. Between them are a pair of Sparta Platforms built into the turf-covered floor below three LED screens that provide graphic displays showing your individual force output in the three phases of a vertical jump, called your Movement Signature, as well as your aggregate score, which combines the results of all three values over time. This is called your Sparta Score. Your Movement Signature can tell you, with a tremendous degree of accuracy, if your training programs are working as intended, what your near-term probability for injury is, and how well-balanced your integrated movement systems are.

Attempting to blend in with the natives, I pulled my rental Subaru into the Sparta parking lot on a bright Wednesday morning with a travel mug full of Starbucks and an iPhone full of questions. Kicking off our conversation, I asked Phil for his thoughts on the concept of fascia training, and if he sees the Sparta Platform being used more for performance optimization or injury reduction.

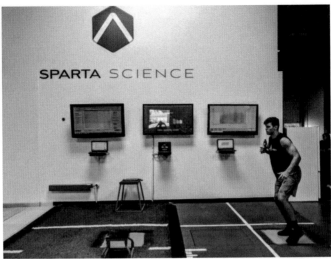

Sparta Science headquarters in Menlo Park, California.
Credit: Johnathon Allen.

"Oh yeah, we're big believers in the fascia system and its role in movement," says Phil. "But one of the challenges in developing constructs is that we tend to want to separate things like performance and injury, when the reality is that they're not separate at all. So you can't just focus on one or the other. At the end of the day, it all comes down to understanding what the data tells us each specific individual needs. Do they need more of a performance approach, or more of an injury resilience approach? For example, we work with the Cavaliers who, in the past, obviously had one of the best players on the planet, and also had a great three-point shooter who wasn't necessarily the most physical.

"So, in that case, one needs more of an injury resilience focus, and one needs more performance. I think one of the big challenges our software solves is providing KPIs that are accurate and reliable.

"An ongoing problem in this field is that people set KPI's that aren't measurable, or at least they're not measurable based on reliable sources of data. Many of them are subjective. Then one of two things happens: Either you don't have any numbers at all to measure your progress, or you get inconsistent or unreliable results that lead to false positives or false negatives. With KPIs, you generally want to know two things: How do you compare against your previous self? And how do you compare against the population—people who play a similar sport or position, are of similar age, etcetera. And that's where the Sparta Scores and the role of our database play in. Another key aspect of KPIs is that they need to be quickly measurable. For example, let's say we use a 40-yard dash. Sure, it's relatively reliable, but the stressfulness of it makes it a poor KPI measurement, because you can only do it once every two to three months, if you want to avoid putting the person at risk for injury."

This is why having a massive source of consistent data makes all the difference. Consider the following math: If you're a strength coach in the NFL with the goal of conditioning your athletes to help reduce ACL injuries, you need data—lots of data—on everything from body type and player position to training programs and recovery protocols. Well, the problem is that, on average, NFL teams only suffer one-and-a-half ACL injuries per year. This means that you'd need more than 63 years of ACL case studies from one team just to achieve the basic minimum for clinical significance. So you really want to aggregate the same kind of data from other teams. The problem is that pro sports teams aren't big on sharing. That's where the Sparta database comes in. Sparta's software makes it possible to anonymously gather and collate force-plate data from every scan entered into the system to create meaningful KPI baselines based on a massive population. Participation in the NFL Combine and other screening events has added even more information to the database, making the Sparta Platform a powerful tool for accurately predicting things like the fact that a linebacker with a Sparta Score above a certain level is five times more likely to start fourteen games next season and, below a certain level, is five times more likely to suffer an ACL injury within the first few.

Just to make sure we're all speaking the same language here, I asked Phil to explain the three phases of a vertical jump as they're measured by Sparta Science, and how those values are used to diagnose injury indicators for different athletes and body types.

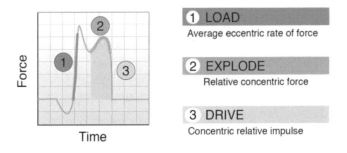

Force signature graph measuring the three phases of a vertical jump. Credit: Sparta Science.

"Sure! 'Load' is the measurement of your eccentric rate of downward force, which has a lot to do with your anterior fascia chain. It tends to be very high in individuals who squat for a living, like linemen and catchers.

In fact, the highest load values we see are in slalom skiers, because they're tucked in that crouch position for like two minutes. So their ability to hold the position is unprecedented in any sport. Load is probably the easiest to improve, because it's really just a matter of getting strong vertically.

"The second phase, 'explode,' is measuring your concentric force—the transition phase, where you're uncoiling. This value tends to be the hardest one to improve, because we believe it's measuring your genetic fast-twitch ability. It can be improved through training, but not nearly as much as the other two values. We see this being very high in individuals who are naturally explosive, with basketball players scoring some of the highest values in this area.

"Then the last value, 'drive,' measures your concentric impulse. It's the only one of the three that multiplies force by time, where the other two divide it. This makes drive the hardest one for most people to understand. You might be inclined to think, why do I want to spend more time producing force? That means I'm slow. But, since it's multiplied, you don't want to have a long time with a low force; you want both of them to be high. We see this in rotational athletes who get to control their tempo and tend not to have to react as much, like pitchers or golfers. They depend more on elastic, fascia-based movements, where they're able to prolong force production more because they're in charge of when it starts and stops. That generates higher drive scores, because they get more control over the whip factor. We tend to see the posterior line of fascia in these athletes being the most extensible and used part of their system.

"They won't have problems doing traditional yoga positions like a downward dog, but their fascia is often a bit too lax in some ways and tightening it up a little is generally a need for them. It's probably part of the reason pitchers have such a problem with high-speed comebacker balls coming right back at them from the hitter. Because they're not reactive athletes."

To paraphrase, this means that a fascia-biased javelin thrower like myself will score high in drive (which I do) while most basketball players (and all but the laziest of kangaroos) will score very high in the explode phase. I asked Phil how he sees a hyper-developed fascia system playing into this dynamic.

"Well, with explosive athletes, I think their fascia is wound so tightly that it acts more like a sensitized trigger finger. Our first partner in this space was Kansas basketball, which might as well be a pro team considering how many of their players go on to the league. And they have so many players with such an outrageous ability to explode that KU's strength and conditioning coach, Andrea Hudy, actually spends a lot of her time working with them on releasing their fascia. She has a whole array of mechanical tools that she uses—like bouncy balls for the feet, golf balls for the heel, and vibration tools for the thighs—because their fascia is so tightly wound that it's not even engaged a lot of the time. And she sees mechanical manipulation in that situation to be just like training. When these players are already so strong and explosive, the question becomes, how do we safely get them to use their fascia more?"

Phil's anecdote about Kansas basketball reminds me of my epiphany watching the Nike tournament kids. So, I asked him if he agreed that their natural explosiveness came from the fact that they spent a lot of their formative years playing a ton of basketball every day.

"Absolutely. Again, a stimulus is a stimulus. It doesn't have to happen in a gym or out on the track. With basketball players, the stimulus tends to be playing a lot of basketball—two hours a day, every day, year-round—so they don't really need much else aside from creating some symmetry in their structure, building up their resilience, and making sure they're tuned up by using things like fascia release."

I find this concept of using targeted mechanotransduction and the mechanical manipulation of fibroblast frequencies to tune the body's fascia system fascinating.

"Yeah, in fact, we often talk about it from a frequency standpoint when we're trying to explain the concept to players—it's like tuning a stereo where you adjust the treble and bass to find the right balance of sound for your body."

And this brings us back to the concept of the Movement Signature and balancing all three values to achieve a high combined output. When I ask Phil about this, he is quick to correct me with an important clarification.

"Well, yes, but what you want is a healthy *imbalance*. Because if all three values are level, then you're probably a little bit good at everything. And, if you're a professional athlete who is a little bit good at everything—but not *great* in anything—you're probably out of a job. What I've been trying to discover—and this is where the database comes in— is how do we push the envelope on how imbalanced you can get based on your specialty without increasing your personal risk for injury.

You'll see players in the NFL, for example, who are really big and super explosive. But they're so imbalanced they can't last more than a few games before they start breaking down. My question is, how do we develop a healthy imbalance that improves an individual's performance without increasing their risk for injury? And it's tracking the difference in the load, explode, and drive that helps you find where that sweet spot is."

Still feeling a bit mystified by it all, I ask what the highest possible Sparta Score is.

"Well, statistically speaking, it's a bell curve. So the middle of that curve is a 50. And every standard of deviation away from the middle of the curve is 10 points. A 60 is one standard of deviation above average. So, the further you get away from 50, the fewer people exist in those categories.

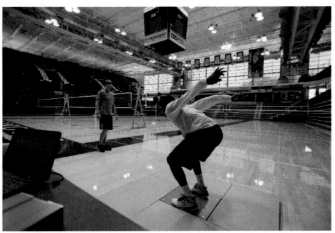

Testing athletes at Santa Clara University with the Sparta Platform. Credit: Sparta Science.

"Exceptional athletes—like your Julio Joneses or your Lebron Jameses of the world—are way out on the tails. There's not really a limit. There are just fewer and fewer people who fall on the outside of the curve distribution."

Right. Math.

"Basically, your aggregate score combines both your performance ability and your injury risk. For example, if I scored 90, 90, 20 on the three values, I wouldn't have a very good Sparta Score—despite the fact that my first two values were very high. That's because the third value's so low, which indicates an increased injury risk. With this approach, it's a matter of laddering up.

"You want to be healthy and balanced, but when you do things to increase your performance, there might be some risk involved. In which case, you would look at what the data says and work to get back to being healthy and balanced. But it's this laddering up process where you really need to monitor risk and performance simultaneously. Ultimately, you're going to be rewarded with a higher aggregate Sparta Score over time."

This approach of using quantifiable data to ladder athletes up makes complete sense to me. I think it's why science-based KPI tools like the Sparta Platform—along with experience and direct observation—are essential for good coaching. Because you need an objective way to quickly assess the person standing in front of you and decide if they're a cheetah or a rhino. So you can understand what training prescriptions that individual really needs. If you're working with a rotational athlete who moves with a lot of drive, doing some light strength

117

work may help them tighten up for better injury resilience and reaction speed, but too much of it will end up inhibiting their top-end performance. Likewise, if you have an explosive kid from Kansas basketball who actually needs some fascia release, and you're constantly putting them under heavy loads with restrictive ranges of motion when they're already tight and stiff, you're actually making them more imbalanced. Noting the standard caveat that generalizations are difficult, I ask Phil the same question I've asked every other expert in this book: What are your general recommendations and prescriptions for whole-system fascia training?

"Well, the way we've approached that question is to work with our client partners to gather information and feedback on different diagnosis and prescription approaches, so we can pull all of this information together to make practical conclusions around the training of fascia and other systems. A good example of this is, by working with one of our partners and looking at the data, we were surprised to discover that doing overhead squats is actually one of the most powerful ways you can improve drive. That realization kind of shattered our previous thinking, because we'd really been pushing a lot of single leg stuff, under the assumption that it was going to improve drive, and overhead squats are a double leg movement. Initially, we thought it was all about the posterior musculature. Which means that if you want to improve drive, you should do things like split-squats, lunges, and RDLs, which all have a very noticeable effect on the musculature and create a ton of delayed-onset soreness that can last up to four days post-exercise. But, when you think about it, an overhead squat makes you go through a full range of motion in both your lower and upper body.

"And when you do it, you don't really get sore, because there's not a lot of weight involved, and it's not just focused on one particular muscle group. To me that was a powerful realization about the significance of fascia. Because when you understand fascia as a connected body-wide system and think about how to best stimulate and activate that system, there's probably no better movement than the overhead squat. It's a huge stimulus that makes fascia tissue more expandable. And I think that highlights the importance of the fascia system, because it speaks to how much the body is connected and how critical fascia is to expressive movement. But it's this ability to classify the effects of different exercises that allows us to prescribe different training approaches for the desired outcome—just like medication."

Again, just to clarify, I'm not trying to sell you Sparta's technology. They recently got backed by $9 million in series-A VC funding and have an unprecedented technology with proven ROI that's being deployed at the highest levels of human performance. They don't need my help. But in my 25-plus years in this industry, Phil is the only guy I've come across who had the personal initiative to go out and develop a data-based screening technology that genuinely changes our understanding of athletic performance and injury reduction and gives us practical tools to measure and improve them. If anything, I'm surprised you probably haven't already heard of him and there isn't a line of coaches, athletes, and team owners climbing over each other to get through Sparta's front door. So I asked him why he thought that was.

"You know, considering how young our company is, I think we're doing pretty great. But when I talk to people who are initially resistant to our technology, I find their main resistance is that they want more freedom around the diagnostic side. And that's a problem, because that's not how health science works. Diagnostics aren't meant to be artistic. They're meant to be standardized. Of course, treatment is a totally different story. That's artistic. Treatment is really where the art of good coaching and good medicine comes into play. But there shouldn't be a lot of flexibility around diagnostics, particularly if you want to predict injuries. Because you need to combine everybody's data to find value in it, and the only way you can do that is if everybody is doing something the same way. If there's a take-home point here, it's that you really need to come at these things with an open mind and look at what the data tells you. Because if you're just focused on your own personal philosophy or worldview, you'll never discover the findings that allow you to be surprised by things like the fascia system."

And that, my friends, is the tectonic sound of a ground-shaking paradigm shift. Or maybe it was an earthquake. I'm not sure. We are in California. Then I just can't resist it anymore and, on my way out the door, shout,

'Thanks Dr. Phil! ... It was real!'

Yup – time to head back to Jersey.

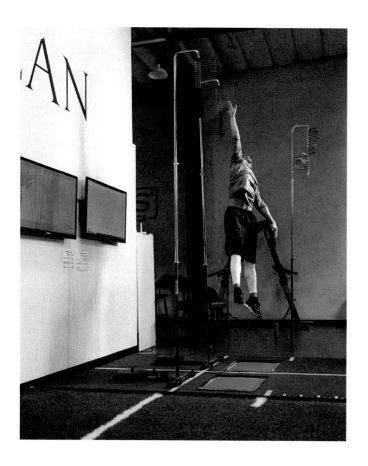

Hacking the Fascia System:
The Power of Proprioception

IF PARADIGM SHIFTS WERE EASY, they'd happen every day. But humans are inherently resistant to change. The illusion that we understand things and that we're in control is probably necessary for us to get out of bed in the morning and confront a world that is in a constant state of motion, variability, and chaos, where the only thing certain is that the Golden State Warriors will win the NBA championship again. But this sense of false confidence, while arguably necessary, is also a trap. Because it keeps us from accepting the fact that we really know very little about how life works, where we came from, and what we are capable of. And this lack of humility holds us back, because you don't get to the next level by staying in your comfort zone and watching reruns. Consider for a moment the possibility that the dots I'm connecting in this book are as game-changing and revolutionary as I think they are—that our bodies operate using a complex integration of balanced systems we have long underappreciated and are only just beginning to understand, thanks to the development of new imaging technologies, research, and diagnostic tools. Now turn that up to 11 and confront the fact that research suggests humans possess latent kangaroo-like superpowers embedded in our biology that we haven't fully unlocked yet, due to our innate tendency to think we already know everything (and because no one invites us to kangaroo parties, which are probably pretty awesome). If this is true, then we're on the verge of an untapped frontier that could radically advance athletic performance, injury reduction, and recovery. These are the thoughts bouncing around my head like a fascia-powered superball as I drive up I-95 from New York City to Westport, Connecticut, to interview Dr. EJ Zebro, co-founder of the TAP Strength Lab sports performance center.

A few things to know about EJ: In addition to being a lifelong soccer player, surfer, and four-time member of the NYC Marathon medical staff, he is also a certified sports chiropractor, therapist, and professional strength coach who developed his own functional movement protocol (TAP™), which has been proven to help improve performance and reduce pain for athletes and patients of all types and ages. Part of the reason I'm going to interview him is that he's also been testing some of OHM's machines at his 3,000-sf functional movement center and performance lab in Westport, and—just like at our facility in Fair Lawn—he's been seeing some impressive results. So I wanted to get his take on why he thought the accommodating resistance modality was so effective and how it fits into the greater concept of fascia training.

"Well, I would say I don't *know* what's happening, but I can tell you what I think is happening," EJ says over lunch at The Spotted Horse Tavern, an upscale horse-themed (!) café and bar built in a renovated circa-1802 federal house in downtown Westport.

"The best description I've heard for the fascia system is that it's like a grapefruit, if you were to cut it in half and suck all the juice out of it: You'd end up with this interconnected 3D web of a matrix that goes all the way through the grapefruit. That's what your fascia system looks like. It's also full of nerve endings, which means that it's a sensory organ that facilitates proprioception.

"Some of the research[27] I've come across recently—which uses ultrasound imaging to analyze fascia tissue—has shown that there is a direct correlation between the increase of fascia thickening and an increase in myofascial pain syndromes. So, for example, if you have someone with chronic low back stiffness, that would imply they had a thickening of fascia in those regions—most likely the deeper layers of fascia tissue that connect directly to the muscle-belly itself—as opposed to the superficial layers. In theory, if you had that person do squat or deadlift movements on the OHM machine, what I feel would happen is that the thickness of their fascia would decrease. The reason that's important is that, as the thickness of your fascia tissue decreases, it increases the soft tissues' ability to glide along one another. This results not only in less stiffness, but also the ability to produce more force. After using these machines over the past year-and-a-half with a wide range of different people, a few things are very clear: Pretty much everyone who uses it claims that they feel like they're somehow gliding through life better, and there is an interesting lack of residual muscle soreness afterwards. The vast majority of responses we get from people is that they feel like they did something the day before—they feel fatigued—but they don't feel sore. To me, that lack of delayed-onset muscle soreness is a result of the fact that their soft connective tissues can glide more easily than they would after experiencing the kinds of compressive forces we deal with when we're doing traditional weight training. Whatever it is, there's definitely something going on there. And for me that something is increased hyaluronic acid—the gliding component of your tissues that provides the viscosity, or 'viscoelasticity,' of fascia."

OK, raise your hand if you already know what hyaluronic acid is. Yup, me neither. So I picked up my phone, checked to make sure we were still recording, and looked it up really fast. Here's the 30-second download: Turns out hyaluronic acid (aka: hyaluronan or HA), is a major component of the extra cellular matrix that is created by a highly specialized type of fibroblast cell. As EJ explained, hyaluronic acid is responsible for the viscosity and sliding action (or lack thereof) between muscles and connective tissues. Your body cycles through a tremendous amount of HA every day. In fact, on average, you have more than 15 grams of it in your tissues right now, and you will rotate through all of it roughly every three days. It essentially determines the viscosity levels of your fascia system that allows you to move smoothly. It also plays major roles in wound healing, inflammation reduction, and cell migration, among other things.

And now, back to our regularly scheduled program.

"When hyaluronic acid is disorganized and not highly concentrated, it turns into a sticky gel that binds fascia tissue together like a kind of glue. But if you can get hyaluronic acid molecules to become more organized and increase their density, they become more like oil, which means they're going to help fascia tissue glide more smoothly over muscle.

"Based on the responses I get from our patients who use the OHM equipment—and extrapolating what I know from fascia manipulation therapy and myofascial techniques in general—I would say it is absolutely effecting their fascia in a way that allows the muscle tissues to recover more quickly and also to produce more power.

I believe that added power comes from increased viscoelasticity. Without that ability to glide, muscle tissues and the soft tissues around them become constricted in their ability to produce force."

I point out that this is in line with the fascia release techniques coach Hudy, at Kansas basketball, uses to help athletes access more of the power stored in their tightly wound tissues.

"Sure!" EJ replies. "One of the techniques I've studied in the last year is a fascia manipulation therapy out of Italy developed by Luigi Stecco. He's developed an extensive practice that really just deals with this one specific form of therapy that's based on using pressure—as opposed to tension—to release fascial restrictions. They've done some very interesting research around why applying pressure to those tissues works. They're looking at the kinetic chains of known meridian lines—such as the posterior chain, anterior chain, lateral lines, and so on. Where it starts to fall off, though, is that they don't have corresponding exercise protocols that go deeply into the global movement patterns of these fascia lines, as well. They'll say, 'Do a clamshell, if there's something going on in the lateral line,' without looking at it in terms of global, closed-chain, multi-joint, multidimensional ranges of motion, which is often what happens with these kinds of techniques. You have a wheelhouse that you're great in, but then you try to be everything to everyone, and it just falls apart."

This brings us back to the problem with generalizing and falling into the trap of "knowing what we know."

Throughout human history, one of the greatest impediments to progress has been the bias of preexisting knowledge and the belief that everything we've been taught by those who've come before us is true—because how could they be wrong? When, in reality, we simply don't know what we don't know. In fact, if we made a list of all the things in the universe that we don't know, it would be pages longer than the list of things we actually do know (and it would start with, "What the hell happened at the end of Lost?"). This warrants pausing our narrative to clarify that, while the name of this book is "Fascia Training," I'm in no way trying to claim that the fascia system can be isolated and trained to the exclusion of the other systems that are all part of the symphony. As many of the experts cited in this book have pointed out, that's impossible. What I'm trying to do is push the needle towards a more accurate understanding of how we think about and train this system, because it's been misunderstood for so long. That's my long-winded way of saying that there isn't just *one* way to train the fascia system. Advances in research and technology are giving us new tools for understanding and developing it, but it's up to us to figure out how to use this information. And that's why I'm trying to understand why three-dimensional isokinetic training modalities like OHM are so effective. I lean into that question more by asking EJ his personal theory.

"It's a good question. And, actually, some of the information I came across in that study we were talking about really helped me think about the answer in new ways. Let me read you part of the transcript and then explain how I think it fits in," EJ replies, as he opens his laptop.

"Ah, here it is: 'Due to different orientations of the collagen fibers in the multiple layers of soft tissue—including the superficial and deep fascia—fascia has a strong resistance to traction or tension. Even when it's exercised in different directions.' So, basically, what they're saying is that if you have, say, a tight hamstring, and you've got tight fascia around the muscles of that hamstring, you could stretch it out all day long, but the fascia is inherently resistant to that sort of traction and tension. The research suggests that it'll respond much better if I take my elbow and jam it into the muscle-belly of your biceps femoris or myotendinous junction of that same line for three minutes. If I do that, and then I have you go back and perform the same active isolation stretch, the fascia is going to respond much better, because we've broken down that scar tissue. I mean, it's just one study. But I think what happens with OHM is that there is an increased amount of time under tension, or time under traction, where your muscles are lengthening and contracting through a full range of motion. But you're doing it in a way that is producing more force, so you're producing more power. You're increasing the traction in the muscles and soft tissues around them in a way that essentially does the same thing fascia manipulation does by sticking an elbow in an area. But it's happening naturally through your body's range of motion, which allows you to get past the breaking point where your fascia tissue would normally not let you go. It's facilitating an easier glide."

Wow, so you're saying that the OHM equipment is somehow hacking the inherent plasticity of fascia tissue and its natural resistance to tension and traction?

"Exactly. And that plasticity part is key—the fact that fascia is resistant to tension. So, sure, you can get more central nervous system input by running faster. But if you have underlying fascia restrictions that are limiting how much tissue is engaged, they are slowing you down. The idea with mechanical manipulation is that by holding elbow pressure on a calf muscle for three minutes you can release the pressure there. And that elbow pressure isn't replicated by moving more quickly, but by moving more slowly. Not because you're neurologically improving the skill of running faster and working on better form, but because you're removing the adhesions that prevented you from reaching full force production. To put it another way, you don't need to go fast to get faster. If you can remove the underlying imbalances in your tissues and sensory nervous system, you'll be able to produce more force, power, and speed throughout your musculoskeletal system."

Is anyone else hearing the distant echo of Tom Myers talking about how "just because you can do something fast doesn't mean you can do it slowly"? Bam—another dot connected.

"I think the key to OHM's accommodating resistance technology is that, no matter who you are, you can exert maximum effort with a tremendous range of motion and personal variability against a responsive form of resistance happening on multiple planes of movement. It almost doesn't make sense. I mean, you keep adding all of these things onto it and think, 'How is that even possible?'"

I know! *Right?* That's why I flew to New York and drove two hours to have this conversation in a boojie bar lined with beautiful, wall-sized photos of running appaloosas. Working in the fitness industry for the past couple of decades, I've pretty much seen all of the gadgets, widgets, and machines that have come out. This is uncharted territory. Listening to EJ extrapolate on why he thinks it works, it occurs to me that he's implying that doing a lot of heavy weight training with limited ranges of motion can actually cause fascia restrictions that ultimately reduce your dynamic force production, not increase it.

"Absolutely! I mean, one of the big problems we see is decreased fascia function from overuse syndrome, which decreases the gliding of your collagen layers and alters your proprioception. A good example of this is saying something like, 'Monday is chest day.' That's an overuse syndrome. Especially if people are lifting the way most people do in Jersey. I can say that—I went to high school in Jersey. I know how I used to lift. Because of that overuse syndrome, you're so tight the next day, you can barely dry your hair. Well, that is altering your proprioception. And if you're trying to perform an activity later that day, but you don't know where you are in time and space, it's going to limit your ability to move. At the same time, we now know that on the physiological level the reason you can't lift your arm over your head is because the collagen layers can't glide like they should. They've become stuck.

"You've turned them into a kind of glue from the repetitive stress you've put on yourself. And I think that's something we don't address enough, or at least I haven't heard it addressed enough: What are the effects of delayed onset muscle soreness in regard to increasing injury risk when you're trying to perform at a high level in a skill or sport? Athletes are often going into a game or event after doing a big leg day, or whatever, and they're still dealing with residual overuse effects, instead of going into that event in a state where everything is gliding smoothly. It's just common sense, right? But no one's really talking about it."I'll give you an example. I lived in Oakland the year of the NBA lockout in the late '90s, and all of the Golden State Warriors were training in the gym I worked at. It was a beautiful 100,000-sf facility called Club One. Guys like Latrell Sprewell, Donyell Marshall, Tony Delk, and a bunch of other amazing players who were in Oakland at the time would drop in to play, and that was pretty much all they did. When they went into the gym, they would stare at the pretty women, pick up the heaviest weight they could do a bicep curl with, bench press a little, get moderately pumped in about seven minutes, and then go play more basketball. I mean, all they were doing was playing basketball. So I think a lot of those athletes skipped the intense repetitive stress stuff, and that allowed them to have these great fascia systems, because their tissues weren't all jacked up from doing the things that a lot of other athletes do to make themselves better."

Again I'm reminded of the Nike tournament kids who became naturally explosive by playing a lot of basketball, the plyometric medicine ball training that helped me excel in college, and the haybale-throwing farm kids who become powerful without ever setting foot in a weight room. And it occurs to me that one of the common themes with all of them is a constant variation of inputs and force vectors—whether it's the rapid running, jumping, and direction-changing of a ball player, or the fact that you can shoot a hundred jump-shots, bounce a hundred med balls, or throw a hundred haybales from the same place, and each one will happen differently every time. Also, all of these examples use natural forms of submaximal resistance that are created by gravity, your own body weight, and variable forces happening on different planes that all activate connective tissues in different ways, as opposed to doing things that involve restrictive motions under heavy loads that create repetitive use syndrome. In theory, this means that using whole-body training techniques with submaximal loads that provide highly variable timing, angle, and force vector inputs can significantly contribute to a more dynamic, well-rounded fascia system. I ask EJ his thoughts on that idea, and if he thinks this variability is part of why OHM's accommodating resistance technology is so effective.

"Sure. I think that's a big part of it. But I would add that the key thing tying it all together is proprioception. Think about a great player like Michael Jordan driving the lane, going up with his right hand and then switching to his left. That guy knew exactly where he was in time and space at all times. Or a guy like Federer. I used to get so annoyed watching him play tennis, because it looked like he wasn't trying hard enough. I wanted him to be out there sweating and grunting, until later when I understood why athletic sustainability is so important. Then I realized that the way he conserves energy and then unleashes it is brilliant. He moves like a dancer. And that's because the fascia system is truly a sensory organ. It has all of these proprioceptive nerve endings bundled up within the tissue, and even more so within the retinaculum that wraps around the tendons in your ankles and wrists. I mean, they're around every joint in your body, but certainly more near the end of your extremities, which is where your proprioceptive organs are. I think that's what you're seeing in these more fascia-based athletes like basketball players. Their proprioception is just incredibly well tuned. And, yes, I think that's related to the variability that comes from doing a jump shot 100 times in a row or the med ball training you were talking about. Those are natural movements that allow you to alter your force production every time, instead of being stuck under 225 pounds and just surviving."

I suggest the idea that repetitive use syndrome essentially drowns out your proprioception in the same way that you become numb to persistent sounds, like a car alarm that won't shut off, or the annoying whine of a squeaky air conditioner fan in your overpriced boutique hotel room. Eventually, your brain just tunes it out.

"I love that analogy!" EJ replies. "You could even take it a step further to emotional intelligence and the cycle of dysfunction that happens when you start repressing your emotions. We've often spoken in our facility about how, if you define yourself by the way you look in the mirror, don't be surprised when you develop the habits of a narcissist—you should've seen the signs. If you just take everything you're feeling and shove it all the way down into the system, it's eventually going to come out. And when it does, it's going to be something like a full-blown labral tear that you thought just happened because you picked something up the wrong way, not because of the thousand times you repressed the fact that you were feeling dysfunctional along the way."

Then I realize that all of the background noises I'd subconsciously tuned out while we were having our discussion have suddenly turned themselves up and come sharply into focus. I can hear the din of a dozen casual lunch conversations mixing with the clatter of flatware, the chirping of cellphones, the rhythmic shaking of the bartender's ice-filled-tumbler, and the distant rumble of traffic. For a moment, it sounds like one groovy, highly variable, constantly evolving free-jazz solo of organized chaos.

And I dig it.

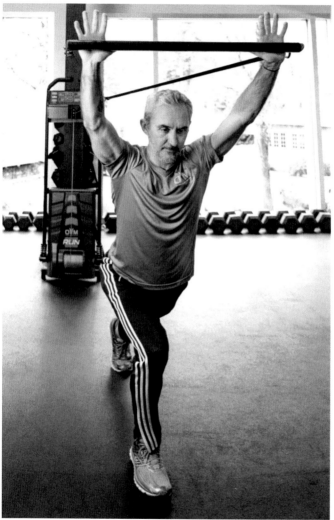

EJ Zebro training on the OHM Run at TAP Strength Lab.

Bill Parisi / Johnathon Allen

Chris Simms: A Case Study in Fascia Training

IT'S A NON-SCIENTIFIC FACT that it's virtually impossible to be both a high school freshman and cool. If you want to pull that trick off growing up in suburban New Jersey, you need swagger, good looks, and mad talent—the kind of talent that makes you not only the starting quarterback of your varsity football team, but one of the top high school quarterbacks in the state before you're even old enough to drive. The kind of talent that makes college recruiters put your name down on a list and then cover it up so no one else sees it. That was Chris Simms. Even at 15, you could tell he had a gifted arm with professional potential. He just needed the right training. And that's why his dad, Super Bowl MVP, Phil Simms, brought him to my first youth training studio in Wykoff, New Jersey, in the middle of his eighth-grade year. As a member of the NY Giants strength and conditioning staff, I'd worked with Phil to help him become one of the top quarterbacks in the NFL. So, as soon as his son was old enough to get serious about sports, he brought him to see me. I tell this story because this relationship gave me the opportunity to train Chris and watch him develop throughout his entire athletic career, from his early formative days as a rock star high school quarterback, to his days at the University of Texas, when they were one of the best college teams in the nation, all the way up to when he became a starting quarterback for the Tampa Bay Buccaneers, where he was almost killed by a savage hit during an early-season game against the Carolina Panthers.

And it occurs to me that Chris is a perfect living case study in whole-system fascia training: What happens when you do it right, what happens when you do it wrong, and how critical it is to injury recovery and rehabilitation. Also, he happens to live about 20 minutes down the road from The Spotted Horse Tavern. So, I decided to drop by while I was in the neighborhood to interview him and see if there were any errant scones laying around that I could use to fuel my drive back to the City.

Quick background reel: When I first met Chris in 1994, he was your typical suburban eighth-grader: a little skinny, a little slow, and a little disinterested in everything. So I put him on a program similar to the one we'd been using in the NFL, the same program that eventually evolved into the Parisi Speed School. A program designed to prime his nervous system, develop his elastic explosiveness, and give him a solid base of strength. We did lots of medicine ball work, plyometrics, speed drills, and other natural techniques to make him fast and dynamic. We did a little light weightlifting to get him stronger and increase his injury resilience—but we never had him lift heavy. We trained him like a martial artist: working slowly at first to develop solid form and movement literacies, then gradually increasing his speed and power as his nervous system tuned up and his connective tissues developed. After Chris started seeing results in a relatively short time, he threw himself into the training program 110 percent, working with me three days a week to get ready for high school tryouts, where he intended to turn some heads. It worked, of course, and he went on to be an outstanding high school athlete at Ramapo High School, playing on both the football and basketball teams. In his junior year on the football team, USA

Today named him National Offensive Player of the Year. After graduating, he joined the Texas Longhorns as a quarterback under legendary coach, Mack Brown, who built one of the top college teams in the nation through a process of savvy scouting and recruiting. But then a curious thing happened. Every time Chris returned home, we would test him. And he always came back slower and less dynamic than when he left. It didn't take me long to figure out why. But Chris is now a color commentator for NBC—which means he gets to talk football and provide his candid opinion for a living—so I'm going to let him explain it.

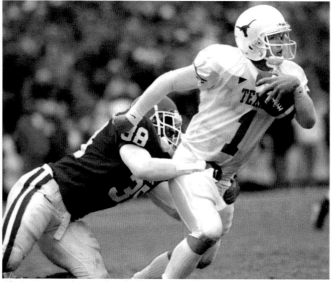

Chris Simms playing for the Texas Longhorns in his freshman year circa 2000. Credit: Tulsa World File.

"Texas had an amazing team with a lot of great players who went on to become first-round draft picks," says Chris. "I didn't start as a freshman, but I played a lot.

"And I truly believe that I opened eyes at Texas before I ever threw a football on the practice field because of all the training and running they had us do in pre-camp. Working with you had made me so fast and explosive in high school that I was probably the most in-shape guy on the Texas football team as a freshman. While I might not have been the fastest guy in the first 100-yard sprint, they would make us run like 20 of them! And on sprints 10 through 20, I was beating guys I had no business beating. The problem was that this approach became too much of the training focus. No disrespect to anyone at Texas, but it was an endurance-based training program back then. You know, the old school method where you just go balls to the wall every day until you're tapping the floor and saying, I quit. I can't do it anymore. We would warm up, do some bag drills, do some cone drills, get really sweaty. And you're thinking, wow, this is a pretty great workout. But then they'd take us out to the track and make us run like sixteen 440s. I mean, when the hell does that ever come into play in football? It was just frying our nervous systems. And because of that, I was just getting beaten down and would gradually become slower and less explosive, until I got back home to restart my training program with you again."

I mention EJ's observations on how overuse syndrome reduces your tissue's ability to glide, ruins your proprioception, and disrupts your nervous system.

"The funny thing about it was that we had some superstar players. We were one of the five best college teams in America, and we had a bunch of top-10 first-round draft picks. We were the real deal. And I started noticing in my junior and senior years that when testing day came, the guys who were the most loyal to being there every day and doing all of the workouts actually tested horribly. And some of the superstars, who played the superstar card and didn't work out all that much because they didn't want to grind themselves into the ground every day, would be the most explosive guys there, because their central nervous systems hadn't been beaten into the freakin' ground for four months. They weren't muscularly fatigued. So, when they ran the 5-10-5, or the 40, or did a max bench press, they would whip everyone else's asses because they weren't totally fatigued."

Fast forward to 2003. Chris is returning home after finishing four years at Texas and has about six weeks to train for the NFL Combine. I'm not going to sugarcoat it—other than still being able to throw a football really well, he was pretty dismal at all the KPIs we'd been measuring him on since he was in eighth grade. His vertical jump had dropped to 20 inches, and he was running the 40 in like 5.2. Yet, oddly, he was bench-pressing 225 pounds like a beast, which is not something quarterbacks typically do.

"What can I say? I prided myself on not being a typical wussy quarterback," Chris says, smiling. "I wanted to be able to move weight. I was benching 225 pounds four or five times a week. If that were something they tested quarterbacks for at the Combine, I probably would have won. But, yeah, I'd lost a lot of my explosiveness in the process. Then you got me back on a training program for the Combine. We worked on explosive starts, running 5-10-5s, doing resisted acceleration work, where I'd be sprinting while you held onto the speed resister. When we retested after 10 days, I was shocked to see performance gains in such a short period of time. When I finally got to the Combine six weeks later, I was jumping more than 31.5 inches and ran the 40 in something like 4.8. I often wonder what would've happened if I hadn't done the Combine and just waited until pro day. How much better would my numbers have been if I'd spent another four weeks doing that specific training before getting tested?"

In retrospect, knowing what I know now and seeing what modern research is revealing about how we actually generate power and speed, I'm surprised at how many things I just intuitively did right when I was starting out as a professional trainer. But this goes back to what Dan Pfaff said about how athletes have a deeply instinctive, often underappreciated sense of what works for them and what doesn't, even if they can't explain why. I originally learned my natural training techniques by being an athlete who just wanted to get better. Also, I think one of the reasons this kind of training works so well is that, in addition to being highly effective, it's also pretty damn fun. And that's one of the secrets to good coaching. Regardless of who you are or what you're training for, if you're trying to achieve your full potential, it's going to involve some hard work. It's going to challenge you at every level. It has to. But if it's not *fun*—if it's *just* work—you're eventually going to burn out and lose interest. Or, at the very least, you're not going to bring the kind of passion that makes inner-city kids play endless basketball on concrete courts under halogen lights long after the sun has gone down and never think of it as a "workout." On the other hand, when it's exciting, challenging, and constantly variable (aka: "fun"), you'll end up doing it for the rest of your life just for the pleasure of being good at it.

Unfortunately, this is the part of the story where it stops being an intriguing case study on the difference between training your fascia system in ways that make you more powerful versus jamming it with overuse syndromes that make you slower, and it becomes a cautionary tale about respecting the critical role fascia plays in injury recovery and rehabilitation.

In 2003, the Buccaneers picked Chris in the third round of the draft under the assumption that he would eventually replace their aging starter, Brad Johnson, who had just led the Bucs to their first-ever Super Bowl victory over the Raiders. In 2005, Chris became the starting quarterback, winning 10 games in a row and leading the Bucs to their first playoff appearance since their Super Bowl win. He was on a roll going into the 2006 season as the team's starter. But I'm going to let Chris tell this part of the story— because he was the one who lived it.

"While we got off to a rough start as a team in 2006, I was personally feeling really good at the beginning of the season. Then, in our fourth game of the season against the Carolina Panthers, I went to throw the ball when I realized I was about to throw an interception. I pulled it back, but the pocket was collapsing. So I decided to throw the ball out of bounds. As I was throwing it, I saw Thomas Davis— who's still playing middle linebacker for the Panthers—running at me full speed. I tried to throw it away before he hit me. But, as I was fully opened up in my throwing motion, Chris Jenkins—who was a 330-pound nose tackle—hit me from behind. I couldn't get out of the way of Davis, and he put his head right into the soft spot of my stomach. And when I say he knocked the wind out of me, I mean he knocked the wind out of me so hard it blew trees down three counties over. I stayed in the game after that, but I could barely call out the next play in the huddle. I was miserable. I actually blacked out at one point. But I somehow managed to lead us on what would have been the game-winning drive until Carolina kicked a 59-yard field goal in the last few seconds to beat us.

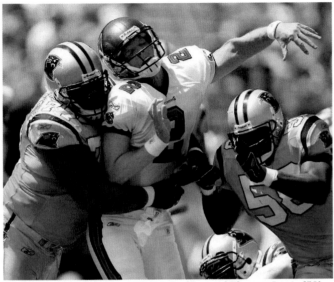

Chris Simms (2) is hit by (77) Kris Jenkins and Thomas Davis (58) in the first quarter during a game between the Tampa Bay Buccaneers vs. Carolina Panthers. Credit: Brendan Fitterer.

"I'd call it a heartbreaker, but it was more of a spleen-breaker. Because what I didn't realize at the time is that I'd ruptured my spleen and was bleeding internally. After the game, they took me to the nearest emergency room and gave me a CAT scan. When the scanner went over my upper body the doctors came running in and were like, 'Oh, Chris, it's really serious! We have to go into emergency surgery right now!' They started cutting my uniform off and medicating me. They actually brought my wife in to say goodbye because they weren't sure I was going to make it. I lost nine pints of blood.

"Thank God, I made it and I'm still here. But after that, I faced a long, hard battle trying to get myself back to being the athlete and person I was before the injury."

One of the problems was that it was 2006, and very few people understood the importance of the fascia system in recovery (with the obvious exception of guys like Stu McGill). We've since learned that moving your body as early as possible after an injury helps prevent the development of long-term fascia adhesions and blockages that limit movement. It's one of the reasons why you now see fewer people wearing restrictive casts and ankle boots. But back then injury recovery was still enshrined in what Tom Myers refers to as the "Temple of Immobility," where recovering patients were directed to rest and not move. This meant that Chris spent months after his surgery avoiding any kind of motion, strain, or activity, which is the kiss of death for a rotational athlete who just had his core cut open.

"I wasn't allowed to do anything strenuous with my core for like five months. They didn't even want me to lift my little girl. After the scar healed, I had to go on a long personal journey searching for doctors and therapists who could help me recover. In the process, I went from having an arm that Jon Gruden said was potentially better than Brett Favre's, to not being able to put enough pace on the ball to break a living room window.

"The fascia in my core was so bound up and restricted that I'd lost the cross-body connection between my upper and lower body that makes you a great thrower. And throwing a ball takes more muscles working cohesively across your entire body than any other motion. But I couldn't create the kinds of opposing forces or generate the level of torque I could before the injury. And I think that's because I was locked down for so long my fascia tissues and muscles completely shut off. I wasn't doing medicine ball throws or the kinds of dynamic exercises that would have allowed me to get the core strength back I needed for twisting my body, creating opposites, and generating force in awkward positions. I was just doing crunches and sit-ups, and the Bucs were like, 'You're looking good, Chris. You can do a crunch again. You should be able to throw the ball 70 yards.' But that wasn't the case at all."

This reminds me of the studies Stu did measuring force production in rats after severing the fascia tissues of their abdominal walls.

"Yeah, right! I get that. Actually, Dr. Anthony Galea up in Canada was one of the first people to show me what was actually going on. He put an ultrasound machine on me while I did crunches and showed me that none of the tissues in my core were even working. He said, 'Sure, you can do a crunch. That's because you're an elite athlete who knows how to recruit other muscles and cheat yourself into making it look like you're doing a crunch.' But the myofascial tissues and muscles around my stomach were basically doing nothing. They were asleep. It wasn't until I started working with specialists, like Greg Roskopf in Denver, that I was able to get back to where I could throw again. And I think the problem is that, in so many situations like this—when a high-performance athlete goes through a serious injury—there's a tendency to jump straight to steps three and four and skip over steps one and two. Then we wonder why the guy who tore his ACL has nine other issues on the same leg in the following years. It's because we tend to get ahead of ourselves and go, 'Hey, he can walk. That's great! Let's start running.' Instead of working on strengthening and restoring the ligaments so that, when he finally sprints, he's using all of his systems the right way and can safely maximize power output again."

Now that Chris covers college and pro sports as a commentator, he's knee-deep in the mix. He has the opportunity to talk to coaches and athletes at every level from aspiring Division One players to accomplished NFL pros. So, I wrap our conversation up by asking him how much understanding he sees of the importance of training the fascia system in conjunction with the musculoskeletal, cardiovascular, and nervous systems, particularly when it comes to injury recovery and avoiding overuse syndrome.

"I think that NFL teams are certainly more advanced now than they've ever been. I'm not saying they're all perfect but, for the most part, head NFL trainers have realized how important it is to train the fascia and nervous systems correctly and how to train players based on their specific position and body type. But in college football—while there are certainly some schools that are moving into the new age—I'd say something like 60 percent of the organizations are still stuck in the old school mentality of, 'We just gotta kill you guys every day until you're crying for mama!' That's definitely still going on, especially at the college level. And, of course, at the high school level, too. But I think it's really a cultural thing. It's just how we were raised. It's how we've always done it. A lot of these ideas—or realizations, really—are relatively new, and people are slow to change."

Driving back to Manhattan in the fading light of another day I imagine a not-so-distant future where modern technology, primal instinct, and the unquenchable desire to win all come together in a flash of athletic glory that, just for a moment, gives us a glimpse of what we're truly capable of, when every instrument in the symphony is rocking out in full unison at full-tilt boogie, and the human kangaroo is finally unleashed.

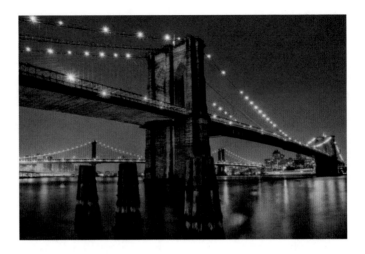

Whatever. You totally knew I was going to bring the kangaroo back. Also, post-rush-hour traffic into the City on a weeknight is surprisingly slow. We have time to kill. Regardless, as I sit in stop-and-go traffic contemplating the untapped capabilities of human athleticism, it occurs to me that I just went on a months-long cross-country road trip from a sailboat off the coast of Maine, to a conference room full of thought leaders outside Vegas, to a startup firm in Silicon Valley, and back to Connecticut, all so I could talk to the different researchers, inventors, and practitioners working at the very edges of their respective fields to advance athletic performance.

I've learned a tremendous amount about the fascia system along the way and gained entirely new perspectives on the new evidence-based science of speed, power, and injury resilience. Then I realize that we're only beginning to understand how important the fascia system really is in all of this—that it's a body-wide sensory organ that plays a much bigger role in movement, force production, proprioception, and injury recovery than we previously recognized.

Thanks to recent advances in imaging technology, research, diagnostic software, and training tools, we're finally reaching a point where we can leave our outdated Newtonian models behind and start knocking on the door of what comes next. But the science is young. And there are still a tremendous number of things we don't know about how it all works. Which means that getting to the next level is going to take a team effort. If you've made it to the end of this book, you probably get that too.

So I encourage you to join me in embracing the cold, uncomfortable reality of the unknown. Use the new tools we have. Ask the hard questions. Find the top experts. Collaborate with them. Look at what the data tells you, and allow yourself to be surprised. Together, we can unlock the next level.

We've only just figured out it's there.

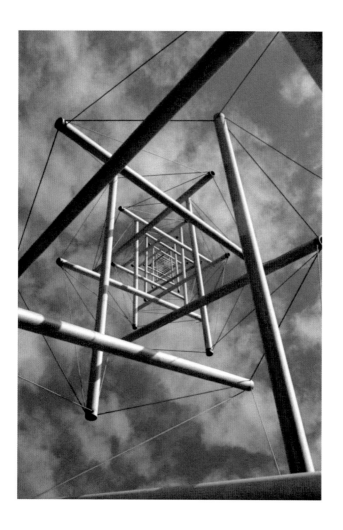

Bill Parisi / Johnathon Allen

Fascia Training: The Matrix

HEY THERE. Thanks for joining us!

What? ... You didn't think I just saw you skim most of the book and jump straight to the last chapter after reading that clever little recap we gave you in the intro?

I'm a coach. I see everything.

It's cool. I do that on Netflix all the time. It's not a terrible strategy. Time is short, and it's a safe bet I'm going to save the best material for the end as a payoff for everyone who sat through the rest of the show (respect to my people in the front row!). That said, you did miss some pretty great stuff. Someone almost died in the last chapter. We went sailing. Stu McGill joked about slicing people up in the name of science. There were a lot of kangaroos. Also a time machine. It got weird. But it was also highly educational. So yeah, maybe give it a spin next time you've got a long flight, or your internet connection is down. In the meantime, you're here now, so grab a seat, buy a hat, and prepare to hold on—it's fourth quarter, slam dunk payoff time, baby!

OK, bring the house lights down. Full disclosure: This was supposed to be a short epilogue chapter where we detailed some specific fascia training techniques you can apply to improve performance and reduce injury based on individual sport, player position, and body type. We are still going to do that, but we've gathered so much great practical information from different experts along the way that we've decided to turn that content into a companion workbook that will hopefully be available soon. As previously mentioned, this is a new science, and we've only just gotten a hold of some of the latest game-changing tools and technologies (i.e. OHM machines, Sparta Platforms, ViPR PROs, etc.). We're currently testing these technologies out at various training facilities and sports performance labs across the country to see what kinds of results we get using the functional, whole-body techniques we've been exploring in this book. We're excited to share those findings with you, so you can use them to inform your own training practices. But we need to do the research and verify the information first. That way, when you say, "show us the data," we can. I have a feeling we're going to be surprised by what we find.

That said, there's one last guy I want to introduce you to before we wrap up, because he probably has more experience applying whole-body fascia training techniques at the professional level than anyone I've ever met. That guy is Todd Wright, an Assistant Coach for the Philadelphia 76ers, as well as their head of strength and conditioning. Before taking that position in 2015, Todd was the strength and conditioning coach for the University of Texas basketball team—yes, the same team that produced players like LaMarcus Aldridge, T.J. Ford, and Kevin Durant. Todd works with basketball players at the top of the top of the game. When I saw him present recently at a PerformBetter conference in Rhode Island, he totally blew my mind. He had tensegrity models. He had Gil Hedley's fuzz video[28]. And he had decades of experience applying these principles to help elite athletes in the most fascia-based sport I can think of. The dude has cut some fresh tracks.

So I pulled him aside after his presentation to thank him for all the great information he provided and dive a little deeper into his training program.

"Thanks, coach! I appreciate that," Todd replied with trademark sincerity. "What do you wanna know?"

Truth be told, I wanted to know a lot of things. Mostly, I wanted to know what he's learned about personalized, fascia-based programming over the past decade (also if he knew what happened at the end of Lost). But I was so impressed with how far ahead of the curve he was, I started out by asking him how he got introduced to the concept of fascia training in the first place.

"Actually, that's an interesting story if you have a few minutes," he replied.

For a guy like Todd, I have all the minutes. Also an iPhone set to record. Let's do this.

"Well coach, like you, I've always been crazy-curious about learning how to help athletes become better. About 20 years ago, I left Clemson University and took over the job at Texas, where I had a core group of guys who were really talented. But two of them had osteitis pubitis, one of them had a shoulder problem, another kid had a knee problem, and I had a kid coming off ankle surgery. But I was coming out of the traditional, old-school world of power-based training. You know, hang cleans, power cleans, push jerks, that sort of thing. And there was a huge gap between my training and knowledge and where I needed to get these guys. So, I started looking around for great physical therapists I could learn from and ended up going to a seminar taught by Gary Gray, called Chain Reaction. How appropriate is that, in regard to the topic of fascia, right? Gary explained to me that applied functional science is the convergence of the biological sciences, the physical sciences, and the behavioral sciences. This experience opened my eyes to the true principles of human movement and how they drive the strategies and techniques we use for coaching. The biggest principles of human movement are that the body is integrated; it functions in an integrated chain reaction transformation; and it's three-dimensional. So, there are three different planes of motion we can move in. If you do an exercise in all three planes of motion, that's called a matrix.

"Another one of the big principles in applied functional science is that the muscles and function of the body are proprioceptively driven. Basically, your muscles and fascia function chain reactively. This chain reaction starts at the subtalar joint, which unlocks your tibia and fibula, and internally rotates your femur, and so on to enable motion. As you move and your foot hits the ground, the proprioceptors in your muscles and fascia react to that movement in the direction that you're going. So, of course, when I started to learn about proprioceptors, I started learning about fascia. Well, if current research is correct, and fascia has five to six times more proprioceptors than muscle, how significant is it in movement and performance? Anyway, by working with Gary, I was able to help a lot of my guys solve issues they'd really been struggling with, and many of them went on to have successful NBA careers. And that experience gave me a new understanding of how the body works. The lens I looked at human movement through really started to evolve and change.

"Fast-forward ten years, and I'm training with my guys. I do a posterior lunge and this loud noise goes off—like the bang of a BB gun. Turns out I had avulsed my adductor longus off of my pelvis. It actually ripped the bone off and it rolled down my leg. And I was thinking, well, I'm lucky. That's the first big injury I've had as a coach. Then about eight months later, I'm in Chicago listening to Thomas Myers speak. He shows us a tensegrity model, and I'm like, what the hell is that thing? He's got these sticks held together with elastic bands and he's telling us, 'This is what your body is.' He shows us how the elastic elements of the tensegrity model are like the ligaments, tendons, and connective tissues that allow our bones—which were the sticks in the model—to free-float in our joint spaces. And I'm thinking, this is fascinating, but if it's true, and we're free-floating in this connected tensional network, I'm screwed. Because I just avulsed my adductor longus, which is a major guy-wire coming off my pelvis. Which means that it's going to create a tensional pull somewhere else in my body, and something is going to end up bothering me somewhere else down the line. Sure enough, another year-and-a-half later, I started having severe neck pain. I stopped sleeping. I couldn't figure it out. So I got an MRI scan, and my neck looked fine. The doctor was looking at the discs, and there was no problem. Well, come to find out, fascia doesn't show up in most MRIs. Then I remembered the learning experience I'd had with Thomas and realized there are no coincidences. So I had some people work on my adductor then follow up along my superficial back line and the spiral line into my neck. Eventually, I got it resolved. After that, I had this totally new perspective on how the body is integrated and held together through our connective tissue matrix, and it just opened my eyes to a whole other realm of learning."

That's when I had my own 'oh-snap!' moment that probably sounded like a BB gun going off, because

I realized Todd was right. If you're paying attention, there are no coincidences. It's not an accident that I'm watching all of these thought leaders come to these conclusions at this point in time like a big cosmic puzzle snapping together. Everything is connected. We're only just now beginning to see how.

This prompted me to ask Todd the million-dollar question, a question his professional and personal experience makes him uniquely qualified to answer: What are some specific things we can do to incorporate this new understanding for better performance and injury prevention?

"Well, first off, you need to realize that the body is three-dimensional, that it moves through three-dimensional space by using the primary drivers of ground reaction, gravity, and mass momentum. Then you need to recognize that fascia is an omni-directional latticework with lines that move in every direction. And, if that is the case, ask yourself why you would train in one sagittal plane of motion using heavy loads, the way a lot of traditional training has been done. Fascia also has plastic remodeling properties that give you the opportunity to change it on a constant basis. Davis's Law states that connective tissue lays downs lines of collagen and reinforcement along lines of stress in the extra-cellular matrix using mechanotransduction—a process where tissues respond to the mechanical forces that we as coaches expose athletes to. This means that it's one of our most trainable systems. And if you change that structure by training it three-dimensionally with sub-maximum loads, at different angles, and different tempos, you can create a more robust foundation for athletes to maneuver through space and win their space in competition."

It occurs to me that we could use Gary Gray's term to describe this and call it "Matrix Training."

"Sure! I get it. You want to come up with a statement that defines your training system. For me, I want our training system to be adaptable. Adaptable to the individual player and also to the needs of the NBA, meaning that I could get a rookie who's had maybe one or two injuries, or I could get a 12-year vet who's had five surgeries.

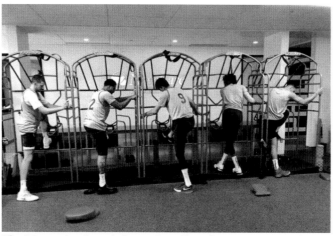

The 76ers using Stretch Cages, that allow them to interactively stretch in an upright position using gravity, ground reaction, and the mass/momentum of their bodies. Credit: Todd Wright/IG.

My goal as a professional strength and performance coach is to allow that athlete to be available for play no matter where they are in their NBA lifecycle. My guys are some of the most gifted athletes in the world, and if they're available for play, we have a high chance of winning games. The question is: How do I learn the stories of their bodies and what they've been through? So when they enter the space, I need to learn their personal stories very quickly.

I need to put them through the core movement patterns required for an NBA game and see if they can transform those movement patterns efficiently and effectively. And if they can't, that needs to be programmed very quickly."

Intrigued, I ask how he quickly diagnoses each individual athlete to identify their personal imbalances, so he can help restore, develop, and enhance their gameplay on the court?

"Right. So if I told you that, I'd have to kill you. And I don't want to do that." (*Why does everyone keep saying that!?*). "Honestly, it's not confidential information. Number one, you really want to listen to the athlete about what bothers them and if they have pain. Then you want to put them through the core movement patterns and observe the three-dimensional functionality of those movements."

Accepting the reality that I may not survive this conversation (I'm doing this for you, team), I press Todd further on what the specific movement patterns are in his program.

"We have eight core movement patterns in our program, and each one is a precursor to the next. There's a squat, a lunge, a leap, a pivot, a jump, a hop, a reach, and a swing. And I can three-dimensionalize each one. So, for example, I can have you squat in all three planes of motion. A squat is a precursor to a jump, right? You have to be able to squat towards your feet to leave the ground. So, if you can't squat in three planes of motion, why would I have you jump in three planes of motion?

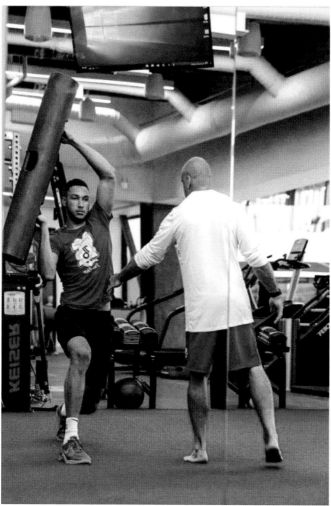

Coach Todd Wright works with Ben Simmons as he does a posterior lunge with a side bend using a ViPR PRO. This movement laterally flexes the core and challenges the body's lateral fascia line in the frontal plane. Source: Todd Wright/IG.

161

"Like you said earlier, basketball is a very three-dimensionally driven game. But there are also a lot of elements in the game that create what we call pattern overload. A good example of pattern overload is that great players will typically have a dominant pivot foot. If you're right-handed, you'll do a lot of things off the left pivot foot and you'll jump off the left foot quite a bit. We know that fascia structures itself along the mechanical lines of stress, so, if you repetitively pivot, load, and jump off your left foot, the lines of stress you put through your left leg verses your right leg are going to be very different. That means the tension in your pelvis will be different, because one side is experiencing more load than the other. You want to create a training system with those pattern overloads in mind, so you can balance those forces within the collagen matrix. In other words, you want to lunge in three directions with submaximal loads; then squat in three planes of motion; then leap in three planes; then pivot in three planes, etcetera, through all eight movement patterns, so you can lay down those lines of stress within the fascia system.

"Our goal is to do that in a consistent, disciplined way every time before we play or practice. We call those accumulation opportunities. And, actually—since you're writing a book about this—that's something worth mentioning. A lot of coaches think that training falls into a place where you need 30 minutes to an hour for a session. My lens is different because of the people I work with. For them, time is a valuable commodity. There's a tendency to think, well he's a pro, he's got plenty of time. But it's not like that. A professional athlete has only a certain amount of time and energy they can allocate to the physical therapists, coaches, and development staff. You get a window in that spot, so you need to be very functionally dense with the strategies you develop to help players create a robust fascia structure. You may get only a six- to eight-minute window where you're able to go through a systematic routine. But, over time, those moments accumulate into movement opportunities that develop and support their fascia system. So when they play, their system is more balanced and they're not reinforcing their pattern overloads. That means we're going to do things like hop on our right leg every day. If you do that five times a day in three different planes of motion, that's 15 jumps daily. And over an 82-game schedule, whatever that number is[29], you accumulate that many opportunities to strengthen that side."

This reminds me of what Tom Meyers said about keeping all of his guy-wires balanced, so his sail doesn't tear in high winds. Identifying pattern overload movements for each specific sport or athlete allows you to help counter those patterns with other movements, so their entire fascia system can share the load.

"Exactly. That means you need to run some diagnostic tests. One of the ways I've been taught to think of the concept of 'transformation' is using the terms 'load' and 'explode.' First, the tissue has to link up and load interactively. But if that tissue can't load because of fascial or muscle restrictions, then you can't explode out of it. So you need to examine a player's ability to load and explode in all three planes through as many movement patterns as possible, so you can diagnose them and create programs tailored to where they are in time."

This prompts me to bring up the Sparta Platform and mention that it's designed to measure those exact metrics and compare them against a deep source of objective data.

"Sure. Of course, there are a lot of diagnostic tools you can use—including video and force plate data—but there's nothing like the eye of an experienced coach who understands movement. What I love about our training system is that it allows me to take my guys through these movement patterns on a daily basis and audit them in three-dimensional movement. When I see a player do a right-leg posterior lunge—and the left-leg lunge doesn't look like the right leg—I can ask them, hey, how are you doing? Does that feel different? And if they say, 'Yeah coach, actually my left front hip is a little tighter,' I know we need to do some work on it."

This makes me wonder if Todd bothers trying to explain the abstract concept of biotensegrity to players who've grown up with a traditional Newtonian perspective of biomechanics and just want to play ball.

"Oh yeah, I have an introductory program for everyone who enters into the program. I show them a tensegrity model—I actually have them all over my office—and explain my goals for them regarding their NBA lifecycle and how I want to help them play at the top of their abilities for a long time. Some get it more easily than others, but it gives me a platform to educate my guys when something goes wrong."

I mention that I find talking to other coaches and players in different sports about the fascia system often comes down to giving them new optics for thinking about human movement and force production.

"Optics is a great word! Because it really comes down to how you see things, right? One of the problems is that the optics in our field haven't been challenged for a long time.

"The truth is that I would probably still be doing a lot of the same things I was doing before I got a hold of these guys who just needed fixing. "But I was really eager to learn a different perspective and get better at what I do, and that allowed me to see these things in new ways. I think the quote that Tom Myer's said once that really rang true for me was along the lines of, 'New discoveries and new techniques will not come from finding new structures, but from looking at known structures in new ways.'"

Inevitably, this prompts me to remember that scene in The Matrix, when Morpheus offers Neo an option between taking the red pill or the blue pill. One lets you go back to your old way of thinking—which is a constructed illusion. The other lets you see the world how it truly is. The catch is that once you do it, you can never go back. On the plus side, you get to move at bullet speed, become an instant Kung Fu master, and wear cool shades everywhere you go (even at night).

So, obviously, it's an easy choice.

And to that I say: Welcome to the Extra-Cellular Matrix. It's a whole new world.

Bill Parisi I Johnathon Allen

Addendum: Fascia Training in Practice

WHAT IS FASCIA TRAINING?

The short answer is that *everything* you do trains the tensional connective tissue network in your body from the time you're born until you've hoed your last row. Also, it's a body-wide sensory organ with tremendous viscoelastic properties that provide the foundation for human speed and power production.

So, the real question is: *how* do you consciously train the fascia system for better speed, power, and injury resilience?

Here are some of the take-home points compiled from each chapter:

Key features of fascia tissue include: viscosity (the ability of your tissues to slide against each other), elasticity (the ability of your tissue to store and release kinetic energy), and plasticity (the ability of your tissue to resist distortion and to reshape itself along lines of stress).

Variability in movement helps reduce overuse syndrome, and pattern overload which inhibits proprioception and increases injury risk. While submaximal loading on multiple planes at different speeds, angles, and tempos using tools like medicine balls, ViPRs, and OHM machines help you develop a healthier, more dimensionally robust collagen matrix resulting in a more balanced whole-body system that allows you to efficiently generate more force.

Developing fascial elasticity is a matter of putting demand on the tissues. This means a foundational element of fascia training is to start out doing movements slowly with proper form and then increasing speed and load as the tissue and nervous system mature and adapt. While significant muscle development can be achieved in a matter of weeks and months, it can take six months to two years to build up balanced body-wide fascial elasticity.

"Fascial elasticity is important, because most tearing injuries occur when connective tissue is stretched faster than it can respond. [...] The muscles typically develop much faster than fascial elasticity, and the greater the imbalance between the two, the higher the chance for injury," – Tom Myers.

"Training for improved elasticity requires short, cyclic, quickly repeated motions, like bouncing, jumping rope, or running on the balls of your feet." - Tom Myers

"Regardless of what you're training for, you need some form of pretraining and conditioning that helps you get all the myofascial units involved to be about the same level of tone. Isolated areas of extra-high tone or low tone predispose an athlete to injury, but when you have an even tone across the body, you'll have the most injury resilience," – Tom Myers.

"Be careful with things like stretching. We don't stretch to create mobility, but that idea is so ingrained in American training culture [...] You can use stretching to tune your fascia system and get it to play with the neurology of the pulse-and-release of elastic energy. But if you stretch fascia elastics away, all you're left with is muscle." – Stu McGill

"It's important not to confuse the tissue adaptation process. For example, if you're lifting with maximal effort one day, and then you go out and try to play golf or throw a javelin the next, you're confusing those tissue adaptations." – Stu McGill

"When I hear people say they're going for 100 percent strength; my response is that your tissues need to *earn* that. You've got to earn the capacity to train at a 100 percent. In fact, I would advise nearly every athlete against it, unless it is pulsed strength." – Stu McGill

"One of the big problems we see is decreased fascia function from overuse syndrome, which decreases the gliding of your collagen layers and alters your proprioception. A good example of this is saying something like, 'Monday is chest day.' That's an overuse syndrome." – EJ Zebro

"I think it's related to the variability that comes from doing a jump shot or throwing a med ball 100 times in a row. Those are natural movements that allow you to alter your force production every time, instead of being stuck under 225 pounds and just surviving." – EJ Zebro

"You need to realize that the body is three-dimensional. It moves through three-dimensional space by using the primary drivers of ground reaction, gravity, and mass momentum. – Todd Wright

"We have eight core movement patterns in our program, and each one is a precursor to the next. There's a squat, a lunge, a leap, a pivot, a jump, a hop, a reach, and a swing. And we three-dimensionalize each one." – Todd Wright

"We'll use ViPRs of anywhere from 24 to 36 pounds to work through the Anatomy Trains lines. We do a posterior lunge for the superficial front line. A lunge matrix with a twist for the functional lines of the body and some of the spiral lines. A squat matrix, where you squat and reach the ViPR away from you so you can load that superficial posterior line. Then, as you reach back, you load the superficial front line. We do a crossover lunge reaching down with the ViPR to get that lateral line. And at the end we'll do some overhead swings and shifts to get into the arm lines." – Todd Wright

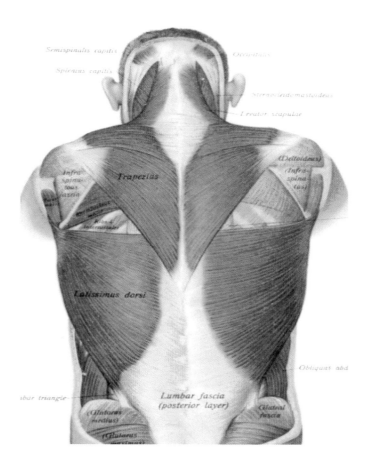

Semispinalis capitis
Splenius capitis
Occipitalis
Sternocleidomastoideus
Levator scapulae
(Deltoideus)
(Infra-spina-tus)
Infra-spina-tous fascia
Trapezius
Latissimus dorsi
Obliquus abd
lumbar triangle
Lumbar fascia (posterior layer)
(Gluteus medius)
(Gluteus maximus)
Gluteal fascia

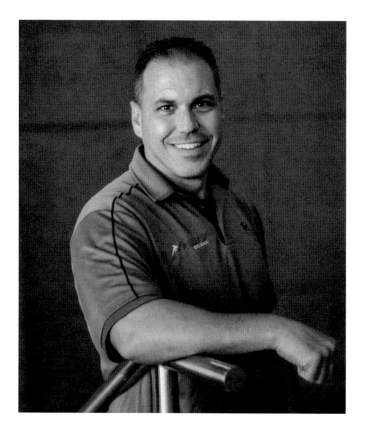

BILL PARISI is the founder and CEO of the Parisi Speed School franchise. With an international team of coaches and facilities in more than 100 locations worldwide, the Parisi Speed School has trained more than 650,000 athletes between the ages of 7 and 18 and produced first-round draft picks in every professional sport—including more than 145 NFL draft picks—and a host of Olympic medalists and champion UFC fighters.

Bill Parisi / Johnathon Allen

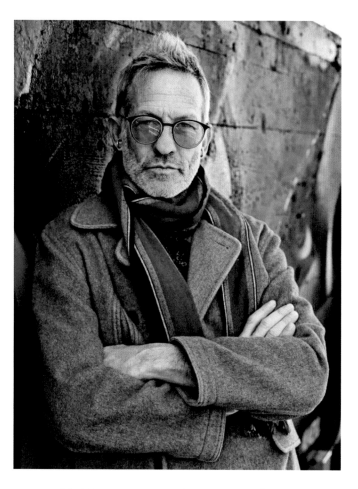

JOHNATHON ALLEN is a writer, photographer, and professional coffee addict based in Portland, Oregon. His work has appeared in *Bicycling*, *Outside*, *Adventure Journal*, *Decline*, and other publications. He is also author of the non-fiction books *Ray's* and *Doppelganger Effect*.

Credits

Cover Design
Giuseppe Lipari | Studio Lipari

Editing
Lisa Wesel | Signal Light

Project Management
Amanda Halliday | Smart Fish Productions

Contact Bill Parisi to organize live events,
speaking engagements, or training seminars:
bparisi@parisischool.com
parisischool.com

Contact Johnathon Allen:
www.allenink.ws
allenink.ws@gmail.com

Press and media inquiries:
parisimediaproductions.com
smartfishproductions.com

Bill Parisi I Johnathon Allen

Resources

Michol Dalcourt
Director of the Institute of Motion
instituteofmotion.com | vipr.com
Twitter: @micholdalcourt

Thomas Myers
Originator of the Anatomy Trains
anatomytrains.com
Twitter: @AnatomyTrains

Dave Schmidt
Founder of OHM Dynamics
OHM.fit

Stuart McGill Ph.D.
Professor emeritus, University of Waterloo
backfitpro.com

Dan Pfaff
Track and Field Coach
Twitter: @pfaffsc

Phil Wagner MD
Founder and CEO of Sparta Science
spartascience.com
Twitter: @DrPhilWagner

EJ Zebro
Founder of TAP Strength Lab
tapstrengthlab.com
Instagram: @dr.ej_zebro

Todd Wright
Founder of Train 4 The Game
train4thegame.com
Instagram: @toddwright_coach

[1] *Helene M. Langevin, MD et al. (2010), Fibroblast Cytoskeletal Remodeling Contributes to Connective Tissue Tension. Journal of Cellular Physiology.*

[2] *Buckminster Fuller (1961), Tensegrity. Portfolio and Art News Annual.*

[3] *Stephen Levin (2015), Tensegrity, The New Biomechanics. Oxford Textbook of Musculoskeletal Medicine. Oxford University Press.*

[4] *D. Ingber (1998), The Architecture of Life. Scientific American.*

[5] *R. Lois Shultz, Rosemary Feitis (1996), The Endless Web: Fascial Anatomy and Physical Reality. North Atlantic Books.*

[6] *Robert Schleip (2017), Fascia as A Sensory Organ: Clinical Applications. Terra Rosa.*

[7] *Todd Ellenbecker (2009), "Effective Functional Progressions in Sport Rehabilitation." Human Kinetics.*

[8] *Aslan Miriyev, Kenneth Stack, Hod Lipson (2017), "Soft Material for Soft Actuators." Nature Communications.*

[9] [9] *R. Kram, TJ Dawson (1998), Energetics and Biomechanics of Locomotion by Red Kangaroos (Macropus rufus). Comp Biochem Physiol.*
http://stripe.colorado.edu/~kram/kangaroo.pdf

[10] *Lewis Sawicki (2009), It Pays to Have a Spring in Your Step. Department of Ecology and Evolutionary Biology, Brown University.*
http://hpl.bme.unc.edu/sawickietal_ESSR_2009_springinstep.pdf

[11] *Y. Kawakami, T. Muraoka, S. Ito, H. Kanehisa and T. Fukunaga (2002), University of Tokyo, Japan. Journal of Physiology.*

[12] *K. Kubo, H. Kanehisa, Y. Kawakami, T. Fukunaga (2001), Effects of Repeated Muscle Contractions on the Tendon Structures in Humans. Eur J Appl Physio.*

[13] *ViPR PRO: vipr.com*

[14] *The multi-disciplinary International Fascia Research Congress, which includes thousands of attendees from over 40 countries, has so far occurred in 2007, 2009, 2012, 2015, and 2018.*

[15] *Huub Maas and Thomas G. Sandercock (2010), Force Transmission between Synergistic Skeletal Muscles through Connective Tissue Journal of Biomedicine and Biotechnology.*
http://dx.doi.org/10.1155/2010/575672

[16] *Helene M. Langevin, MD, and Peter A. Huijing, PhD (2009), Communicating About Fascia: History, Pitfalls, and Recommendations. Massage Bodywork.*
https://www.ncbi.nlm.nih.gov/pmc/articles/PMC3091474/

[17] *Wolffe, 1892,*
https://www.ncbi.nlm.nih.gov/pubmed/8060014

[18] [18] *Y. Kawakami, T. Muraoka, et al. (2002), "In vivo Muscle Fiber Behavior During Counter-Movement Exercise in Humans Reveals a Significant Role for Tendon Elasticity." Journal of Physiology.*

[19] *https://www.instagram.com/p/BlzErJ7hufS/*

[20] *Jordan M. Joy, Ryan P. Lowery, Eduardo Oliveiera De Souza, Jacob M. Wilson (2013), Elastic Bands As a Component of Periodized Resistance Training. Journal of Strength and Conditioning Research.*

[21] *Peter G. Weyand, Deborah B. Sternlight, Matthew J. Bellizzi, and Seth Wright (2000), Faster Top Running Speeds are Achieved with Greater Ground Forces Not More Rapid Leg Movements. Journal of Applied Physiology.*
https://doi.org/10.1152/jappl.2000.89.5.1991

[22] *Peter G. Weyand, Rosalind F. Sandell, Danille N. L. Prime, and Matthew W. Bundle (2010), The Biological Limits to Running Speed are Imposed from The Ground Up. Journal of Applied Physiology.*

[23] *Kenneth P. Clark, Peter G. Weyand (2014), Are Running Speeds Maximized with Simple-Spring Stance Mechanics? Journal of Applied Physiology. https://doi.org/10.1152/japplphysiol.00174.2014*

---

[24] *Stephen H.M. Brown, Stuart M. McGill (2010), Transmission of Muscularly Generated Force and Stiffness Between Layers of the Rat Abdominal Wall. SPINE Vol. #34.*

[25] *Stuart M. McGill (2004), Ultimate Back Fitness and Performance. Wabuno Publishers.*
Available from www.backfitpro.com

[26] *R. McNeill Alexander (2003) Principles of Animal Locomotion. Princeton University Press.*

[27] *Martina Zügel, Paul William Hodges, Robert Schleip, Thomas Findley (2018), Fascial Tissue Research in Sports Medicine: From Molecules to Tissue Adaptation, Injury and Diagnostics.*

[28] *https://youtu.be/_FtSP-tkSug*

[29] *1,230*

Made in the USA
Middletown, DE
04 March 2022